Keto Baking

Easy Keto Diet Sweet and Savory Baking Recipes including Bread, Buns, Cookies, Bars, Cakes, Muffins, and More

David Martin

Efforts were made to ensure that the information in this book is accurate and complete. However, the author and the publisher do not warrant the accuracy of the information, text, and graphics contained within the book due to the rapidly changing nature of science, research, known and unknown facts, and the internet. The author and the publisher do not hold any responsibility for errors, omissions, or contrary interpretation of the subject matter herein. This book is presented solely for motivational and informational purposes.

The recipes provided in this book are for informational purposes only and are not intended to provide dietary advice. A medical practitioner should be consulted before making any changes in diet. Additionally, recipes' cooking times may require adjustment depending on age and quality of appliances. Readers are strongly urged to take all precautions to ensure ingredients are fully cooked to avoid the dangers of foodborne illnesses.

The recipes and suggestions provided in this book are solely the opinions of the author. The author and publisher do not take any responsibility for any consequences that may result due to following the instructions provided in this book. The nutritional information for recipes contained in this book is provided for informational purposes only. This information is based on the specific brands, ingredients, and measurements used to make the recipe, and therefore the nutritional information is an estimate, and in no way is intended to be a guarantee of the actual nutritional value of the recipe made in the reader's home. The author and the publisher will not be responsible for any damages resulting in your reliance on the nutritional information. The best method to obtain an accurate count of the nutritional value in the recipe is to calculate the information with your specific brands, ingredients, and measurements.

ISBN: 9798699407804

Printed in the United States

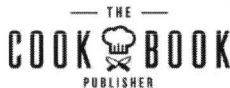

—— THE ——
COOK BOOK
PUBLISHER
www.thecookbookpublisher.com

CONTENTS

INTRODUCTION

It's no mystery why we all love to bake so much. All that whipping and beating is worth it when you march towards the oven with a big smile on your face to bake a mouthwatering masterpiece.

The traditional approach to baking is to prepare breads, rolls, cakes, muffins etc. using wheat flour and a few flours from other grains. But the world of baking has now expanded to suit all types of healthy diets, including the revolutionary Keto Diet. The ketogenic diet has taken every continent on this planet by storm. More and more people are becoming aware of the health benefits of adopting a high-fat, low-carb diet. Not only does it keep extra weight off your body, it ensures that you stay ideally nourished to keep serious diseases at bay. The Keto Diet has become a secret weapon for total fitness and wellness.

Baked goods are truly mesmerizing and simply mouthwatering. If you have decided to adopt the healthy Keto Diet lifestyle, that does not mean saying goodbye to the heavenly aromas and perfect textures of baked items. Without breaking any Keto Diet rules, you can experience the joy of baking and eating all types of breads, cookies, muffins and cakes. All you need is the right book in your hand, and this is it.

KETO BAKING ESSENTIALS

Baking is magic, and baking with low-carb, high-fat Keto Diet ingredients is the ultimate magic. With few smart swaps, you can convert any regular baking pantry into a keto-baking pantry. Prepare your pantry with these essential keto-baking ingredients for easy baking and lots of smiles to come.

Keto Flours

Almond Flour

Made from blanched ground almonds, almond flour is a popular swap for all-purpose flour, whole wheat flour, etc. It is rich in healthy fats, and more importantly, it is low in carbohydrates. You can use it to make bread, cookies, muffins, etc. It is readily available in any nearby supermarket.

Coconut Flour

Made from ground dried coconut meat, coconut flour is another popular swap for regular baking flours. If you prefer a coconut-based taste in your baked goods over a nutty taste, then you should choose coconut flour instead of almond flour. Recipes made with coconut flour are fluffy in texture and have a moist consistency. Coconut flour is a rich source of fiber as well as healthy fats, and it's low in carbohydrates too.

Coconut and almond are the most commonly used flours when it comes to keto baking, but there are a couple of others you can also consider

Flaxseed Meal

Flaxseed meal is also known as linseed meal. Just like coconut and almond flour, it is low in carbohydrates and rich in fiber as well as omega–3 fatty acids. It is rarely used as a standalone flour but is mostly mixed with almond or coconut flour for preparing cookies, muffins, bread, etc. with a variety of textures and improved nutritional density.

Psyllium Husk Powder

Less common but sometimes used in keto bread recipes as a binding agent, psyllium husk powder is a low-carb, high-fiber powder that makes an ideal replacement for xanthan gum and also eggs (if you prefer egg-less baking). However, try to minimize its consumption if you have a sensitive digestive system—it is also used as a laxative agent!

Sweeteners

Since keto recipes can't have sugar in them, how do you sweeten them? Here are three of the most popular choices

Erythritol

Produced through natural fermentation in fruits, erythritol is a zero-carb sugar alcohol that is most commonly available in granular form. Erythritol is is used quite frequently in all types of keto baking recipes. The only problem with using erythritol is that it can make recipe mixtures too dry. To preserve the liquid balance, you can use it in combination with stevia drops or simply add water until you get the desired consistency.

Monk Fruit

Monk fruit is a natural sweetener sourced from a plant. Just like erythritol, monk fruit is a zero-carb sugar substitute.

Stevia

Stevia a very popular plant-based sweetener that is available as both drops and granules. It's easy to replace one with another in any recipe because a conversion chart (stevia granules to stevia drops and vice versa) comes with the pack.

Fats

Oil, Ghee, and Butter

When it comes to cooking fats, you don't need to change much for keto baking. You can freely use butter and ghee in all keto baking recipes.

If you prefer dairy-free baking, use ghee, which is clarified butter to which all its milk solids have been removed.

As for oils, coconut and olive are the most popular choices. Both are keto-friendly oils that are known for their healthy composition of fats and other nutrients.

Leavening Agents

Baking Soda and Baking Powder

Many people wonder if they can use baking soda and baking powder without increasing carbohydrate values. The good news is that baking soda does not contain any carbs at all; it can be freely used for all types of keto baking recipes.

Baking powder does contain carbs, but only a minimal 1.3 grams per teaspoon.

With a wide range of low-carb keto baking recipes to explore, you do not have to give up your favorite bread, cookies, muffins, cakes, and bars. You can satisfy your cravings without compromising on maintaining a healthy low-carb lifestyle. This exclusive book on keto baking covers all types of delectable baked goods to infuse life into your ketogenic diet plan. From soft bread to aromatic muffins, each recipe covered in this book comes with simple baking instructions to suit beginners as well as kitchen experts.

Get ready to grab an apron and learn to bake the best of keto baking recipes at home. Let's get started!

SAVORY BAKED GOOD RECIPES

Breads, Buns, and Rolls

Coconut Cream Bread

*Yields 1 loaf | Prep. time 15 minutes |
Cooking time 40 minutes*

Ingredients
⅓ cup water, heavy cream or coconut milk
6 eggs
⅓ cup olive/coconut oil or butter
½ cup ground flaxseed
½ cup coconut flour
1 tablespoon baking powder
1 teaspoon xanthan gum
2 tablespoons granulated sweetener
½–1 teaspoon ground cinnamon
½ teaspoon salt

Directions
1. Preheat the oven to 375°F (190°C). Line an 8×4-inch loaf pan with parchment paper.
2. Beat the eggs in a mixing bowl. Add the oil/butter and water/cream/milk. Mix well.
3. To another mixing bowl, add the coconut flour and remaining ingredients. Mix well.
4. Combine the mixtures until smooth and without visible lumps.

5. Add the mixture to the loaf pan. Smooth the top with a spatula or spoon. Sprinkle some sesame seeds on top.
6. Bake for 40–45 minutes until the top turns golden brown. Check by inserting a toothpick; if it doesn't come out clean, bake for a few more minutes and repeat.
7. Remove pan from oven and let bread cool completely on a wire rack.
8. Slice and serve fresh.

Nutrition (per slice)
Calories 122, fat 9 g, carbs 4 g, dietary fiber 3 g
Protein 4 g, sodium 127 mg

Walnut Nut Bread

Serves 10 slices | Prep. time 10 minutes |
Cooking time 40 minutes

Ingredients

2 tablespoons psyllium husk powder
½ teaspoon salt
½ cup coconut flour
1 tablespoon baking powder
4 eggs
2 tablespoons apple cider vinegar
¼ cup olive/coconut oil
1 cup walnuts chopped
½ cup boiling water (if needed)

Directions

1. Preheat the oven to 350°F (175°C). Line an 8×4-inch loaf pan with parchment paper.
2. Add the baking powder, coconut flour, psyllium husk powder, and salt to a mixing bowl. Mix well.
3. In another bowl, beat the eggs. Add the apple cider vinegar and oil. Mix well.
4. Combine the mixtures and mix well until no visible lumps remain.
5. Add the walnuts and mix again.
6. Optionally mix in the water (in batches) until you get a smooth batter.
7. Shape into a dough. Add to the loaf pan. Smooth the top with a spatula or spoon.
8. Bake for 35–40 minutes until the top turns golden brown. Check by inserting a toothpick; if it doesn't come out clean, bake for a few more minutes and repeat.
9. Remove pan from oven and let bread cool completely on a wire rack.
10. Slice and serve fresh.

Nutrition (per slice)
Calories 188, fat 16 g, carbs 7 g, dietary fiber 4 g
Protein 5 g, sodium 389 mg

Mixed Seed Bread

Yields 1 loaf | Prep. time 15 minutes |
Cooking time 35 minutes

Ingredients
½ cup coconut flour
2 tablespoons flaxseed flour
1 tablespoon chia seeds
¼ cup sunflower seeds
¼ cup pumpkin seeds
2 tablespoons coconut oil
2 eggs
4 egg whites
1 tablespoon apple cider vinegar
2 tablespoons psyllium husk powder
½ teaspoon salt
1 tablespoon baking powder
½ cup boiling water

Directions
1. Preheat the oven to 350°F (175°C). Line an 8×4-inch loaf pan with parchment paper.
2. Add the baking powder, coconut flour, psyllium husk powder, salt and flaxseed flour to a mixing bowl. Add all of the seeds, but reserve some seeds for later use. Mix well.
3. In another bowl, beat the eggs. Add the oil and apple cider vinegar. Mix well.
4. Combine the mixtures until smooth and without visible lumps.

5. Mix in some water until you get the desired consistency.
6. Add the mixture to the loaf pan. Smooth the top with a spatula or spoon. Sprinkle the reserved seeds on top.
7. Bake for 30–35 minutes until the top turns golden brown. Check by inserting a toothpick; if it doesn't come out clean, bake for a few more minutes and repeat.
8. Remove pan from oven and let bread cool completely on a wire rack.
9. Slice and serve fresh.

Nutrition (per slice)
Calories 116, fat 7 g, carbs 9 g, dietary fiber 6 g
Protein 5 g, sodium 413 mg

Oregano Cauliflower Bread

Yields 1 loaf | Prep. time 15 minutes |
Cooking time 90 minutes

Ingredients
½ cup almond flour or coconut flour
1 egg
2 egg whites
1 teaspoon apple cider vinegar
1 large cauliflower, trimmed and cut into florets
1 tablespoon pumpkin seeds
2 tablespoons cream cheese
1 teaspoon sea salt
1 teaspoon baking soda
Oregano, paprika, cayenne pepper, etc. for seasoning

Directions

1. Preheat the oven to 350°F (175°C). Grease an 8×4-inch loaf pan with coconut/olive oil or cooking spray.
2. In a blender, blend the cauliflower florets into fine crumbs or a grain-like consistency. Do not over-blend.
3. Add the cauliflower crumbs and almond flour to a mixing bowl. Mix well.
4. In another bowl, beat the egg whites until soft peak forms. Set aside.
5. In another bowl, beat the whole eggs; add the apple cider vinegar and cream cheese. Mix well. Add the egg whites and mix again.
6. Combine the mixtures until smooth and without visible lumps.
7. Mix in seasoning to taste.
8. Add the mixture to the loaf pan. Smooth the top with a spatula or spoon. Sprinkle the sea salt and pumpkin seeds on top.
9. Bake for 10 minutes; reduce temperature to 300°F (150°C).
10. Bake for 50–60 minutes until the top turns golden brown. Check by inserting a toothpick; if it doesn't come out clean, bake for a few more minutes and repeat.
11. Remove pan from oven and let bread cool completely on a wire rack.
12. Slice and serve fresh or store in the refrigerator for up to four days.

Nutrition (per slice)

Calories 44, fat 2.5 g, carbs 3.5 g, dietary fiber 1.5 g
Protein 3 g, sodium 19 mg

Garlic Cheese Bread

Yields 1 loaf |Prep. time 15 minutes |
Cooking time 45 minutes

Ingredients
1 teaspoon baking powder
2 cups almond flour
½ teaspoon salt
½ cup butter, softened
½ teaspoon xanthan gum
6 eggs
1 tablespoon parsley flakes
½ tablespoon oregano flakes
2 tablespoons garlic powder
1 cup cheddar cheese or cheese blend, shredded

Directions
1. Preheat the oven to 355°F (176°C). Line an 8×4-inch loaf pan with parchment paper.
2. Add the xanthan gum, baking powder, salt and almond flour to a mixing bowl. Mix well.
3. In another bowl, beat the eggs. Add the butter. Mix until well blended and frothy.
4. Combine the mixtures. Add the parsley, garlic, cheese and oregano.
5. Combine until smooth and without visible lumps.
6. Add the mixture to the loaf pan. Smooth the top with a spatula or spoon.
7. Bake for 45 minutes until the top turns golden brown. Check by inserting a toothpick; if it doesn't come out clean, bake for a few more minutes and repeat.
8. Remove pan from oven and let bread cool completely on a wire rack.
9. Slice and serve fresh.

Nutrition (per slice)
Calories 108, fat 9 g, carbs 2.5 g, dietary fiber 0.5 g
Protein 4.5 g, sodium 162 mg

Zucchini Walnut Bread

*Yields 1 loaf | Prep. time 15 minutes |
Cooking time 55 minutes*

Ingredients
5 large eggs
1 teaspoon vanilla extract
½ cup butter, softened
¾ cup granulated sweetener
¼ cup coconut flour
1½ cups almond flour
½ teaspoon xanthan gum
4 teaspoons baking powder
1 teaspoon cinnamon
½ cup chopped walnuts
½ teaspoon salt
2 cups grated zucchini, squeezed to remove excess water

Directions
1. Preheat the oven to 350°F (175°C). Line a 9x5 loaf pan with parchment paper.
2. Add the baking powder, cinnamon, almond flour, coconut flour, xanthan gum and salt to a mixing bowl. Mix well.
3. In another bowl, beat the eggs. Add the sweetener and butter. Mix until well blended and fluffy.
4. Mix in the vanilla extract.
5. Combine the mixtures until smooth and without visible lumps.
6. Mix in the grated zucchini.

7. Add the mixture to the loaf pan. Smooth the top with a spatula or spoon.
8. Bake for 50–55 minutes until the top turns golden brown. Check by inserting a toothpick; if it doesn't come out clean, bake for a few more minutes and repeat.
9. Remove pan from oven and let bread cool completely on a wire rack.
10. Slice and serve fresh.

Nutrition (per slice)
Calories 171, fat 15 g, carbs 5 g, dietary fiber 3 g
Protein 5 g, sodium 318 mg

Almond Bread

Yields 1 loaf | Prep. time 10 minutes |
Cooking time 30 minutes

Ingredients
3 teaspoons baking powder
1½ cups almond flour
6 large eggs, separated
¼ cup butter, melted
¼ teaspoon cream of tartar (optional)
6 drops liquid stevia (optional)
1 pinch salt

Directions
1. Preheat the oven to 375°F (190°C). Grease an 8×4-inch loaf pan with some butter.
2. Beat the egg whites in a mixing bowl. Add the cream of tartar. Mix until soft peaks form.

3. Add the butter, salt, baking powder, stevia, yolks and ⅓ of the egg whites to a blender or food processor and blend until smooth.
4. Add the remaining egg whites and blend until smooth.
5. Add the mixture to the loaf pan. Smooth the top with a spatula or spoon.
6. Bake for 30 minutes until the top turns golden brown. Check by inserting a toothpick; if it doesn't come out clean, bake for a few more minutes and repeat.
7. Remove pan from oven and let bread cool completely on a wire rack.
8. Slice and serve fresh.

Nutrition (per slice)
Calories 90, fat 7 g, carbs 2 g, dietary fiber 0.7 g
Protein 3 g, sodium 43 mg

Broccoli Cheddar Bread

Yields 1 loaf | Prep. time 15 minutes |
Cooking time 30 minutes

Ingredients
¾ cup raw broccoli florets, chopped
1 cup shredded cheddar cheese
3½ tablespoons coconut flour
2 teaspoons baking powder
1 teaspoon salt
5 eggs, beaten

Directions
1. Preheat the oven to 350°F (175°C). Grease an 8×4-inch loaf pan with coconut/olive oil or cooking spray.
2. Add all the ingredients except for the eggs to a mixing bowl. Mix well.
3. In another bowl, beat the eggs.
4. Combine the mixtures until smooth and without visible lumps.
5. Add the mixture to the loaf pan. Smooth the top with a spatula or spoon.
6. Bake for 30–35 minutes until the top turns golden brown. Check by inserting a toothpick; if it doesn't come out clean, bake for a few more minutes and repeat.
7. Remove pan from oven and let bread cool completely on a wire rack.
8. Slice and serve fresh.

Nutrition (per slice)
Calories 90, fat 6 g, carbs 2 g, dietary fiber 1 g
Protein 6 g, sodium 342 mg

Zucchini Sun Dried Tomato Bread

Yields 1 loaf | Prep. time 10 minutes |
Cooking time 60 minutes

Ingredients
½ cup unsweetened almond milk
¾ cup salted butter, melted
4 eggs
½ cup shredded zucchini
2 cups almond flour
¼ cup coconut flour
2 tablespoons sun-dried tomatoes, chopped
4 teaspoons baking powder
1 teaspoon granulated sweetener
½ teaspoon dried parsley
¼ teaspoon garlic powder
½ teaspoon dried oregano
½ teaspoon xanthan gum
1¼ teaspoon salt
½ cup shredded Asiago cheese

Directions
1. Squeeze the shredded zucchini to remove excess water.
2. Preheat the oven to 350°F (175°C). Grease a 9×5-inch loaf pan with coconut/olive oil or cooking spray.
3. Add all of the dry ingredients except for the cheese to a mixing bowl. Mix well.
4. In another bowl, beat the eggs. Add the almond milk, zucchini, butter and tomatoes. Mix well or blend in a blender or food processor.
5. Combine the mixtures until smooth and without visible lumps.
6. Mix in the Asiago cheese.

7. Add the mixture to the loaf pan. Smooth the top with a spatula or spoon.
8. Bake for 50–60 minutes until the top turns golden brown. Check by inserting a toothpick; if it doesn't come out clean, bake for a few more minutes and repeat.
9. Remove pan from oven and let bread cool completely on a wire rack.
10. Slice and serve fresh.

Nutrition (per slice)
Calories 262, fat 23 g, carbs 3 g, dietary fiber 1 g
Protein 8 g, sodium 533 mg

Bacon Cheddar Bread

Yields 1 loaf | Prep. time 15 minutes |
Cooking time 45 minutes

Ingredients
1 tablespoon baking powder
7 ounces bacon
1½ cups almond flour
2 large eggs
¼ cup butter, melted
⅓ cup sour cream
1 cup cheddar cheese, shredded

Directions
1. Add the bacon to a medium saucepan or skillet and cook over medium heat until crisp evenly and evenly brown. Drain over paper towel and crumble.
2. Preheat the oven to 300°F (150°C). Grease an 8×4-inch loaf pan with coconut/olive oil or cooking spray.

3. Add the almond flour and baking powder to a mixing bowl. Mix well.
4. In another bowl, beat the eggs. Add butter and sour cream. Mix well.
5. Combine the mixtures until smooth and without visible lumps.
6. Mix in the crumbled bacon and cheddar cheese.
7. Add the mixture to the loaf pan. Smooth the top with a spatula or spoon. Add more cheddar cheese on top if desired.
8. Bake for 45 minutes until the top turns golden brown. Check by inserting a toothpick; if it doesn't come out clean, bake for a few more minutes and repeat.
9. Remove pan from oven and let bread cool completely on a wire rack.
10. Slice and serve fresh.

Nutrition (per slice)
Calories 306, fat 26 g, carbs 5 g, dietary fiber 2 g
Protein 14 g, sodium 174 mg

Rosemary Focaccia Bread

Yields 1 loaf | Prep. time 10 minutes |
Cooking time 20–25 minutes

Ingredients
2 tablespoons fresh rosemary, chopped
1 tablespoon baking powder
¾ teaspoon salt
1 cup almond flour
⅓ cup coconut flour
½ teaspoon garlic powder
2 large eggs
2 large egg whites
½ cup olive oil
¼–½ cup water
Coarse sea salt and rosemary leaves

Directions
1. Preheat the oven to 325°F (160°C). Line a baking sheet with parchment paper and grease it with coconut/olive oil or cooking spray.
2. Add the rosemary, baking powder, almond flour, coconut flour, salt and garlic powder to a mixing bowl. Mix well.
3. In another bowl, beat the whole eggs and egg whites. Add the olive oil. Mix well.
4. Combine the mixtures into a smooth dough without visible lumps.
5. Place the dough on the baking sheet and roll it into a 9×12-inch rectangle.
6. Dimple the dough with your fingertips; sprinkle rosemary leaves and sea salt on top.
7. Bake for 20–25 minutes until the edges firm up and turn golden brown.
8. Remove pan from oven and let bread cool completely on a wire rack.

9. Slice into rectangles and serve fresh.

Nutrition (per serving)
Calories 174, fat 15 g, carbs 5 g, dietary fiber 2.5 g
Protein 6 g, sodium 209 mg

Hot Dog Buns

Serves 4 | Prep. time 10 minutes | Cooking time 12 minutes

Ingredients
2 teaspoons baking powder
½ teaspoon baking soda
1 cup almond flour
3 tablespoons Parmesan cheese
¼ teaspoon onion powder
½ teaspoon garlic powder
1 pinch salt
2 tablespoons unsalted butter
¾ cup grated mozzarella cheese
1 teaspoon white vinegar
2 eggs

Directions
1. Preheat the oven to 375°F (190°C). Line a baking sheet with parchment paper and grease it with coconut/olive oil or cooking spray.
2. Add the Parmesan, almond flour, garlic powder, onion powder, baking powder, baking soda and salt to a mixing bowl.
3. Mix well; add the mozzarella and mix again. Add the butter on top.
4. Microwave for 20–30 seconds until cheese melts. Mix well.

5. In another bowl, beat the eggs. Set aside 1 tablespoon and add the remainder to the flour mixture. Mix well.
6. Mix in the vinegar.
7. Divide into 4 parts and shape each into a log.
8. Place them on the baking sheet. Brush on top with the reserved egg wash.
9. Bake for 12–minutes until the top turns golden brown.
10. Remove sheet from oven and let buns cool completely on a wire rack.
11. Serve fresh.

Nutrition (per serving)
Calories 350, fat 30 g, carbs 7 g, dietary fiber 3 g
Protein 15.5 g, sodium 342 mg

Cauliflower Buns

Serves 4 | Prep. time 15 minutes | Cooking time 15 minutes

Ingredients
½ cup mozzarella cheese, shredded
¼ cup cheddar cheese, shredded
¾ pound cauliflower, cut into florets
1 egg
¼ cup almond flour

Directions
1. Preheat the oven to 400°F (200°C). Grease a baking sheet with coconut/olive oil or cooking spray.
2. Cook the cauliflower florets in boiling water until tender; drain and set aside.
3. Add all of the ingredients (including the cauliflower) to a blender or food processor.

4. Blend for 30–40 seconds until well combined.
5. Add the mixture to the baking sheet in 4 scoops. Gently press to shape into buns.
6. Bake for 12–15 minutes until the top turns golden brown.
7. Remove sheet from oven and let buns cool completely on a wire rack.
8. Serve fresh.

Nutrition (per serving)
Calories 151, fat 10 g, carbs 6 g, dietary fiber 2.5 g
Protein 10 g, sodium 22 mg

Classic Keto Buns

Serves 4 | Prep. time 20 minutes | Cooking time 25 minutes

Ingredients
¼ cup hot water
3 medium egg whites
1 medium egg
¼ cup coconut flour
¼ cup almond flour
1 teaspoon baking powder
1 tablespoon psyllium husk powder
Sesame or other seeds

Directions
1. Preheat the oven to 355°F (176°C). Line a baking sheet with parchment paper and grease it with coconut/olive oil or cooking spray.
2. Add the dry ingredients to a mixing bowl. Mix well or blend with a blender or food processor.
3. In another bowl, beat the egg and egg whites. Add the hot water. Mix well.

4. Combine the mixtures until smooth and without visible lumps.
5. Divide into four parts and shape into buns.
6. Place the buns on the baking sheet. Sprinkle seeds on top.
7. Use a knife to make crisscross cuts in the top.
8. Bake for 25 minutes until the top turns golden brown.
9. Remove the baking sheet from the oven and let the buns cool completely on a wire rack.
10. Serve fresh.

Nutrition (per serving)
Calories 109, fat 5.5 g, carbs 8.5 g, dietary fiber 5 g
Protein 7 g, sodium 18 mg

Mozzarella Burger Buns

Serves 6 | Prep. time 10 minutes | Cooking time 12 minutes

Ingredients
3 large eggs
3 cups almond flour
2 cups shredded mozzarella
4 ounces cream cheese
1 teaspoon salt
2 teaspoons baking powder
4 teaspoons butter, melted
Sesame seeds
Dried parsley

Directions
1. Preheat the oven to 400°F (200°C). Line a baking sheet with parchment paper and grease it with coconut/olive oil or cooking spray.

2. Add the almond flour, baking powder and salt to a mixing bowl. Mix well.
3. In another bowl, beat the eggs. Add the cream cheese and mozzarella. Mix well.
4. Combine the mixtures until smooth and without visible lumps.
5. Divide into six parts and press gently to shape into buns.
6. Place the buns on the baking sheet. Brush with butter and sprinkle sesame seeds and parsley on top.
7. Bake for 10–12 minutes until the top turns golden brown.
8. Remove the baking sheet from the oven and let the buns cool completely on a wire rack.
9. Serve fresh.

Nutrition (per serving)
Calories 323, fat 26 g, carbs 6 g, dietary fiber 2 g
Protein 17 g, sodium 641 mg

Garlic Cheese Dinner Rolls

Yields 8 | Prep. time 10 minutes | Cooking time 25 minutes

Ingredients
1½ cups almond flour
2 large eggs, beaten
1 teaspoon garlic powder
1 teaspoon Italian seasoning
1 teaspoon baking powder
2 cups shredded mozzarella cheese
2 ounces full-fat cream cheese

Garlic Topping
2–3 cloves garlic, minced
2 tablespoons butter
1 tablespoon Italian seasoning or minced parsley
¼ cup Parmesan or cheddar cheese (optional)

Directions
1. Preheat the oven to 350°F (175°C). Grease a baking pan with some butter or coconut oil.
2. Add the cream cheese and mozzarella to a mixing bowl. Microwave for 20–30 seconds until cheese melts. Mix well.
3. Add the baking powder, almond flour, eggs, garlic powder and Italian seasoning.
4. Combine until smooth and without visible lumps.
5. Divide dough into 8 balls and shape into rolls.
6. Place rolls on the baking pan.
7. To another bowl, add the butter, parsley and garlic; whisk well.
8. Brush mixture on top of balls; sprinkle with more cheese on top (optional).
9. Bake for 25 minutes until the top turns golden brown. Check by inserting a toothpick; if it doesn't

come out clean, bake for a few more minutes and repeat.

10. Remove pan from oven and let cool completely on a wire rack.
11. Serve fresh.

Nutrition (per roll)
Calories 269, fat 23 g, carbs 6 g, dietary fiber 2 g
Protein g, sodium 239 mg

Classic Dinner Rolls

Yields 6 | Prep. time 10 minutes | Cooking time 15 minutes

Ingredients
2 eggs, separated
1¾ ounces almond flour
1¾ ounces cream cheese
½ teaspoon baking powder
¼ teaspoon cream of tartar
Salt to taste
2 tablespoons olive oil

Directions
1. Preheat the oven to 360°F (180°C). Grease a baking pan with coconut/olive oil or cooking spray.
2. Add the cream cheese to a mixing bowl. Microwave for 20–30 seconds until cheese melts. Add the olive oil and mix well to emulsify evenly.
3. Add the almond flour, baking powder and salt; whisk well.
4. Add the egg yolk and continue to mix.
5. In another bowl, beat the egg whites. Add the cream of tartar. Mix well.

6. Combine the mixtures until smooth and without visible lumps.
7. Divide into 6 parts and shape into rolls.
8. Place rolls on the baking pan.
9. Bake for 12–15 minutes until the top turns golden brown. Check by inserting a toothpick; if it doesn't come out clean, bake for a few more minutes and repeat.
10. Remove pan from oven and let cool completely on a wire rack.
11. Serve fresh.

Nutrition (per roll)
Calories 141, fat g, carbs 2 g, dietary fiber 1 g
Protein 4 g, sodium 63 mg

Rosemary Flaxseed Dinner Roll

Yields 6 | Prep. time 15 minutes | Cooking time 15 minutes

Ingredients
1 cup almond flour
6 tablespoons ground flaxseed
1 cup mozzarella cheese, shredded
1 ounce cream cheese, softened
½ teaspoon baking powder
½ teaspoon chopped thyme
1 teaspoon chopped rosemary
1 tablespoon butter, melted
1 large egg, whisked
2 cloves garlic, minced

Directions

1. Preheat the oven to 400°F (200°C). Line a baking sheet with parchment paper.
2. Add the cream cheese and mozzarella to a mixing bowl. Microwave for 20–30 seconds until cheese melts. Mix well.
3. Add the almond flour, baking powder and flaxseed.
4. Add half of the herbs and mix well.
5. In another bowl, beat the eggs.
6. Combine the mixtures into a smooth dough without visible lumps.
7. Roll into a log shape and divide into six parts. Roll each part into a ball.
8. Place balls on the baking sheet.
9. Add the butter, garlic and remaining herbs to a mixing bowl. Mix well.
10. Brush half of the mixture over the balls.
11. Bake for 12–15 minutes until the top turns golden brown. Check by inserting a toothpick; if it doesn't come out clean, bake for a few more minutes and repeat.
12. Remove pan from oven and let cool completely on a wire rack.
13. Serve rolls fresh with the remaining butter mixture on top.

Nutrition (per roll)

Calories 200, fat 16 g, carbs 5.5 g, dietary fiber 3.5g
Protein 8 g, sodium 89 mg

Bagels

Classic Keto Bagels

Serves 8 | Prep. time 15 minutes | Cooking time 25 minutes

Ingredients
3 cups mozzarella cheese, shredded
2 ounces cream cheese
2 cups almond flour
1 tablespoon baking powder
3 large eggs, lightly beaten
3 tablespoons bagel seasoning of your choice

Directions
1. Preheat the oven to 400°F (200°C). Line two baking sheets with parchment paper.
2. Add the mozzarella and cream cheese to a mixing bowl. Microwave for 20–30 seconds until cheese melts. Mix well.
3. Add the baking powder and almond flour to a mixing bowl. Mix well.
4. Mix in the melted cheese.
5. In another bowl, beat 2 eggs.
6. Combine the mixtures until smooth and without visible lumps.
7. Divide into 8 parts. Roll each part into a ball. Press your finger in the center of each ball to create a hole, then move it in a circular motion to stretch into a bagel shape.
8. Place the bagels on the baking sheets. Beat the remaining egg and brush on top; sprinkle with bagel seasoning.
9. Bake for 20–25 minutes until the top turns golden brown.

10. Remove from oven and let cool completely on a wire rack.
11. Serve fresh.

Nutrition (per serving)
Calories 212, fat 17 g, carbs 4 g, dietary fiber 1 g
Protein 15 g, sodium 310 mg

Pecan Pumpkin Bagels

Serves 6 | Prep. time 15 minutes | Cooking time 15 minutes

Ingredients
2 eggs, beaten
2 cups almond flour
2 ounces cream cheese
1½ cups shredded mozzarella cheese
1–2 tablespoons granular sweetener
1 tablespoon baking powder
1 tablespoon pumpkin pie spice
⅓ cup pumpkin puree
3 tablespoons crushed pecans (divided)
1 tablespoon olive oil

Topping
1 tablespoon granular sweetener
¼ teaspoon cinnamon
4 ounces cream cheese, softened

Directions
1. Preheat the oven to 400°F (200°C). Line a baking sheet with parchment paper.
2. Add the mozzarella and cream cheese to a mixing bowl. Microwave for 20–30 seconds until cheese melts. Mix well.

3.   Add the eggs and continue to mix.
4.   Add the baking powder, almond flour, pumpkin pie spice, sweetener and pumpkin puree to a mixing bowl. Mix well.
5.   Mix in 2 tablespoons of the pecans.
6.   Divide into 6 parts. Press your finger in the center of each ball to create a hole, then move it in a circular motion to stretch into a bagel shape.
7.   Place the bagels on the baking sheet. Brush with olive oil and sprinkle with the remaining pecans.
8.   Bake for 10–15 minutes until the top turns golden brown.
9.   Remove from oven and let cool completely on a wire rack.
10. Serve fresh.

Nutrition (per serving)
Calories 456, fat 39 g, carbs g, dietary fiber 6 g
Protein 17 g, sodium 505 mg

Super Seed Bagels

Serves 4 | Prep. time 15 minutes | Cooking time 30 minutes

Ingredients
½ teaspoon baking powder
1 tablespoon psyllium husk powder
1 medium egg
½ cup coconut flour
2 tablespoons butter, melted
1 tablespoon chia seeds
2 tablespoons sunflower seeds
1 cup boiling water

Directions

1. Preheat the oven to 400°F (200°C). Line a baking sheet with parchment paper.
2. Add the coconut flour, psyllium husk powder and baking powder to a mixing bowl. Mix well.
3. In another bowl, beat the eggs. Add the butter. Mix well.
4. Mix in the sunflower and chia seeds.
5. Combine the mixtures until smooth. Add the boiling water in batches and continue to mix until no visible lumps remain.
6. Divide into 4 parts. Press your finger in the center of each ball to create a hole, then move it in a circular motion to stretch into a bagel shape.
7. Place the bagels on the baking sheet.
8. Bake for 15 minutes; turn over and bake for 15 more minutes until the top turns golden brown.
9. Remove from oven and let cool completely on a wire rack.
10. Serve fresh.

Nutrition (per serving)

Calories 209, fat g, carbs 6 g, dietary fiber 1 g
Protein 7 g, sodium 112 mg

Cinnamon Bagels

Serves 16 | Prep. time 15 minutes | Cooking time 10 minutes

Ingredients
1½ cups shredded mozzarella cheese
2 ounces cream cheese
1 teaspoon vanilla extract
1 egg, beaten
1 cup almond flour
3 tablespoons coconut flour
3 tablespoons powdered or granulated sweetener
2 teaspoons baking powder

Coating
1 tablespoon melted butter
1 tablespoon granulated sweetener
2 teaspoons cinnamon

Directions
1. Preheat the oven to 400°F (200°C). Line a baking sheet with parchment paper.
2. Add the mozzarella and cream cheese to a mixing bowl. Microwave for 20–30 seconds until cheese melts. Mix well.
3. Add the almond flour, coconut flour, sweetener and baking powder to a mixing bowl. Mix well.
4. Combine the mixtures and mix well.
5. In another bowl, beat the eggs. Mix in the vanilla extract.
6. Add to the flour mixture. Mix well until no visible lumps remain.
7. Refrigerate for 30 minutes.
8. Divide into 16 parts. Press your finger in the center of each ball to create a hole, then move it in a circular motion to stretch into a bagel shape.

9. Place the bagels on the baking sheet. Brush on top with butter.
10. Add the cinnamon and granulated sweetener to a mixing bowl. Mix well.
11. Roll each bagel in the cinnamon mixture and place on the baking sheet.
12. Bake for 10 minutes until the top turns golden brown.
13. Remove from oven and let cool completely on a wire rack.
14. Serve fresh.

Nutrition (per serving)
Calories 95, fat 7 g, carbs 3 g, dietary fiber 1 g
Protein 5.5 g, sodium mg

Cauliflower Bagels

Serves 6 | Prep. time 20 minutes | Cooking time 22 minutes

Ingredients
¼ cup superfine almond flour
¼ cup coconut flour
4 cups cauliflower, finely chopped
2 cups part skim mozzarella cheese, shredded
4 large eggs
2 teaspoons baking powder
Bagel seasoning of your choice

Directions
1. Preheat the oven to 400°F (200°C). Line a baking sheet with parchment paper.
2. Add the cauliflower, baking powder, almond flour, coconut flour and mozzarella to a mixing bowl. Mix well.
3. In another bowl, beat 3 eggs.
4. Combine the mixtures until smooth and without visible lumps.
5. Divide into 6 parts. Press your finger in the center of each ball to create a hole, then move it in a circular motion to stretch into a bagel shape.
6. Place the bagels on the baking sheets. Beat the remaining egg and brush on top; sprinkle with bagel seasoning.
7. Bake for 20–22 minutes until the top turns golden brown.
8. Remove from oven and let cool completely on a wire rack.
9. Serve fresh.

Nutrition (per serving)
Calories 231, fat g, carbs 11 g, dietary fiber 4 g
Protein 17 g, sodium 331 mg

Garlic Bagels

Serves 6 | Prep. time 15 minutes | Cooking time 15 minutes

Ingredients
2 teaspoons xanthan gum (optional)
6 eggs
⅓ cup butter or ghee, melted
½ cup coconut flour, sifted
½ teaspoon salt
½ teaspoon baking powder
1½ teaspoons garlic powder

Directions
1. Preheat the oven to 400°F (200°C). Grease a 6-hole doughnut pan with coconut/olive oil or cooking spray.
2. Add the coconut flour, xanthan gum and baking powder to a mixing bowl. Mix well.
3. In another bowl, beat the eggs. Add the garlic powder, salt and butter. Mix well.
4. Combine the mixtures until smooth and without visible lumps.
5. Pour into the doughnut pan.
6. Bake for 15 minutes until the top turns golden brown.
7. Remove from oven and let cool completely on a wire rack.
8. Serve fresh.

Nutrition (per serving)
Calories 202, fat 16 g, carbs 7 g, dietary fiber 4 g
Protein 7 g, sodium 397 mg

Breadsticks and Crackers

Classic Keto Breadsticks

Yields 6–8 | Prep. time 15 minutes |
Cooking time 12 minutes

Ingredients
1 teaspoon baking powder
¼ teaspoon salt
½ teaspoon oregano
½ teaspoon dried basil
½ teaspoon garlic powder
½ teaspoon dried thyme
3 tablespoons coconut flour
1 cup almond flour
Olive oil

Wet Ingredients
2 teaspoons apple cider vinegar
1 egg
1 tablespoon ground flaxseed mixed with 2 tablespoons water

Directions
1. Preheat the oven to 350°F (175°C). Line a baking sheet with parchment paper.
2. Beat the eggs in a mixing bowl. Mix in the apple cider vinegar and flaxseed.
3. Add the baking powder, salt, both of the flours and all of the herbs to a mixing bowl. Mix well.
4. Make a well in the center and pour in the egg mixture. Mix well.
5. Knead for 1–2 minutes until you get a smooth dough.

6. Refrigerate for 10–15 minutes.
7. Divide dough into 6–8 pieces. Roll each to form a breadstick.
8. Place on the greased baking sheet. Brush with olive oil.
9. Bake for 10–12 minutes until breadsticks are crisp and top is evenly brown.
10. Remove from oven and let cool completely on a wire rack.
11. Serve fresh.

Nutrition (per breadstick)
Calories 84, fat 5 g, carbs 4.5 g, dietary fiber 2 g
Protein 3 g, sodium 148 mg

Italian Seasoned Breadsticks

Yields 24 | Prep. time 15 minutes | Cooking time 15 minutes

Ingredients
1 tablespoon psyllium husk powder
3 tablespoons cream cheese
2 cups (8 ounces) mozzarella cheese, shredded
1 large egg
1 teaspoon baking powder
¾ cup almond flour

Seasoning
1 teaspoon salt
1 teaspoon pepper
2 tablespoons Italian seasoning

Directions

1. Preheat the oven to 400°F (200°C). Grease a baking sheet with coconut/olive oil or cooking spray.
2. Beat the eggs in a mixing bowl. Add the cream cheese. Mix well.
3. Add the almond flour, psyllium husk and baking powder to a mixing bowl. Mix well.
4. Add the mozzarella to a mixing bowl. Microwave for 20–30 seconds until cheese melts. Mix well.
5. Add to the egg mixture and mix well. Add the flour mixture.
6. Combine the mixtures into a smooth dough without visible lumps.
7. Roll the dough flat between two pieces of wax paper.
8. Slice into 24 breadsticks.
9. Place on the greased baking sheet.
10. Combine all of the seasoning ingredients in a bowl. Sprinkle evenly over breadsticks.
11. Bake for 13–15 minutes until breadsticks are crisp and top is evenly brown.
12. Remove from oven and let cool completely on a wire rack.
13. Serve fresh.

Nutrition (per 4 breadsticks)

Calories 238, fat 19 g, carbs 5.5 g, dietary fiber 3 g
Protein g, sodium 189 mg

Super Cheesy Breadsticks

Yields 24 | Prep. time 15 minutes | Cooking time 15 minutes

Ingredients
1 tablespoon psyllium husk powder
3 tablespoons cream cheese
2 cups (8 ounces) mozzarella cheese, shredded
1 large egg
1 teaspoon baking powder
¾ cup almond flour

Topping
¼ cup Parmesan cheese, shredded
3 ounces cheddar cheese, shredded
1 teaspoon garlic powder
1 teaspoon onion powder

Directions
1. Preheat the oven to 400°F (200°C). Grease a baking sheet with coconut/olive oil or cooking spray.
2. Beat the eggs in a mixing bowl. Add the cream cheese. Mix well.
3. Add the almond flour, psyllium husk and baking powder to a mixing bowl. Mix well.
4. Add the mozzarella to a mixing bowl. Microwave for 20–30 seconds until cheese melts. Mix well.
5. Add to the egg mixture and mix well. Add the flour mixture.
6. Combine the mixtures into a smooth dough without visible lumps.
7. Roll the dough flat between two pieces of wax paper.
8. Slice into 24 breadsticks.
9. Place on the greased baking sheet.

10. Combine all of the cheese topping ingredients in a bowl. Sprinkle evenly over the breadsticks.
11. Bake for 13–15 minutes until breadsticks are crisp and top is evenly brown.
12. Remove from oven and let cool completely on a wire rack.
13. Serve fresh.

Nutrition (per 4 breadsticks)
Calories 314, fat 24.5 g, carbs 6.5 g, dietary fiber 2.5 g
Protein 18 g, sodium 81 mg

Garlic Herbed Breadsticks

Yields 6 | Prep. time 20 minutes | Cooking time 12 minutes

Ingredients
⅓ cup coconut flour
½ cup almond flour
1 teaspoon baking powder
2 cups mozzarella cheese, shredded
3 tablespoons cream cheese
1 teaspoon salt
1 tablespoon garlic powder
1 egg
2 tablespoons chopped parsley

Spread
1 teaspoon garlic powder
1 teaspoon oregano
Pinch of chopped parsley
2 tablespoons butter

Directions

1. Preheat the oven to 400°F (200°C). Grease a baking sheet with coconut/olive oil or cooking spray.
2. Beat the eggs in a mixing bowl.
3. Add the garlic powder, almond flour, coconut flour, parsley, baking powder and salt to a mixing bowl. Mix well.
4. Add the mozzarella and cream cheese to a mixing bowl. Microwave for 40–60 seconds until cheese melts. Mix well.
5. Add to the egg mixture and mix well. Add the flour mixture.
6. Combine the mixtures into a smooth dough without visible lumps.
7. Divide dough into 6 pieces. Roll each to form a breadstick.
8. Place on the greased baking sheet.
9. Bake for 12 minutes until breadsticks are crisp and top is evenly brown.
10. Remove from oven and let cool completely on a wire rack.
11. Add all of the garlic spread ingredients to a mixing bowl. Microwave for 20 seconds. Mix well.
12. Brush the breadsticks with garlic butter; serve fresh.

Nutrition (per breadstick)
Calories 145, fat 9 g, carbs 8 g, dietary fiber 4.5 g
Protein 6 g, sodium 428 mg

Cinnamon Breadsticks

Yields 24 | Prep. time 15 minutes | Cooking time 18 minutes

Ingredients
1 tablespoon psyllium husk powder
3 tablespoons cream cheese
2 cups (8 ounces) mozzarella cheese, shredded
1 large egg
1 teaspoon baking powder
¾ cup almond flour

Topping
6 tablespoons granular sweetener
2 tablespoons cinnamon
3 tablespoons butter, melted

Directions
1. Preheat the oven to 400°F (200°C). Grease a baking sheet with coconut/olive oil or cooking spray.
2. Beat the eggs in a mixing bowl. Add the cream cheese. Mix well.
3. Add the almond flour, psyllium husk and baking powder to a mixing bowl. Mix well.
4. Add the mozzarella to a mixing bowl. Microwave for 20–30 seconds until cheese melts. Mix well.
5. Add to the egg mixture and mix well. Add the flour mixture.
6. Combine the mixtures into a smooth dough without visible lumps.
7. Roll the dough flat between two pieces of wax paper.
8. Slice into 24 breadsticks.
9. Place on the greased baking sheet.
10. Combine all of the cinnamon topping ingredients in a bowl. Sprinkle evenly over the breadsticks.

11. Bake for 13–15 minutes until breadsticks are crisp and top is evenly brown.
12. Remove from oven and let cool completely on a wire rack.
13. Serve fresh.

Nutrition (per serving)
Calories 291, fat 24.5 g, carbs 7 g, dietary fiber 4 g
Protein g, sodium 63 mg

Mozzarella Crackers

Yields 40 | Prep. time 15 minutes | Cooking time 8 minutes

Ingredients
⅛ teaspoon garlic powder
⅛ teaspoon salt
1 large egg yolk
½ cup mozzarella cheese, shredded
⅓ cup finely ground almond flour

Directions
1. Preheat the oven to 425°F (220°C). Line a baking sheet with parchment paper.
2. Add the mozzarella, garlic powder, almond flour and salt to a mixing bowl. Microwave for 20–30 seconds until cheese melts. Mix well.
3. Beat the egg yolk in a mixing bowl. Combine with the flour mixture to form a smooth dough.
4. Roll the dough flat between two pieces of wax paper.
5. Poke holes in it with a fork.
6. Slice into 1-inch squares.
7. Place on the greased baking sheet.
8. Bake for 5–6 minutes; flip.

9. Bake for 2 more minutes until crackers are crisp and top is evenly brown.
10. Remove from oven and let cool completely on a wire rack.
11. Serve fresh.

Nutrition (per 5 crackers)
Calories 55, fat 4 g, carbs 1.5 g, dietary fiber 0.5 g
Protein 3 g, sodium 81 mg

Garlic Herb Crackers

Yields 40 | Prep. time 20 minutes | Cooking time 15 minutes

Ingredients
1 egg
¼ cup coconut flour
¼ cup almond flour
2 teaspoons garlic powder (divided)
1 tablespoon Italian herb mix
1 clove garlic
1 teaspoon salt (divided)
¼ cup butter
1¾ cups mozzarella cheese, shredded
2 tablespoons sour cream

Directions
1. Preheat the oven to 400°F (200°C). Line a baking sheet with parchment paper.
2. Add the mozzarella to a mixing bowl. Microwave for 20–30 seconds until cheese melts. Mix in the sour cream and mix well.
3. Add the herb mix, almond flour, coconut flour and 1 teaspoon of the garlic powder to a mixing bowl.

4. In another bowl, beat the eggs. Mix with the cheese mixture.
5. Mix in the flour mixture to make a smooth dough.
6. Refrigerate for 10–15 minutes.
7. Roll the dough flat between two pieces of wax paper.
8. Poke holes in it with a fork.
9. Slice into 1-inch squares.
10. Place on the greased baking sheet.
11. Add the melted butter, garlic clove, remaining garlic powder, and ½ teaspoon of the salt to a bowl.
12. Microwave for 3–5 minutes until butter melts. (You can also use a saucepan for this step.)
13. Brush the crackers with the butter mixture. Sprinkle with the remaining salt.
14. Bake for 6–7 minutes; flip.
15. Bake for 6–7 more minutes until crackers are crisp and top is evenly brown.
16. Remove from oven and let cool completely on a wire rack.
17. Serve fresh.

Nutrition (per 5 crackers)
Calories 112, fat 8 g, carbs 4 g, dietary fiber 1.5 g
Protein 6.5 g, sodium 317 mg

Flaxseed Crackers

Yields 20 | Prep. time 20 minutes | Cooking time 25 minutes

Ingredients
2 tablespoons Parmesan cheese
¾ cup ground flaxseed
⅓ cup finely ground almond meal flour
1½ tablespoons herb mix (oregano, rosemary, thyme, etc.)
½ cup water
¼ teaspoon salt
⅛ teaspoon pepper
1 tablespoon olive oil

Directions
1. Preheat the oven to 380°F (190°C). Line a baking sheet with parchment paper.
2. Add the almond flour, ground flaxseed, herbs and seasonings to a blender or food processor and blend well.
3. Add the olive oil and continue to blend.
4. Pour in the water and mix into a smooth dough.
5. Roll the dough flat between two pieces of wax paper.
6. Poke holes in it with a fork.
7. Slice into 1-inch squares.
8. Place on the greased baking sheet.
9. Bake for 18–25 minutes until crackers are crisp and top is evenly brown, flipping crackers halfway through.
10. Remove from oven and let cool completely on a wire rack.
11. Serve fresh.

Nutrition (per 2 crackers)
Calories 85, fat 6.5 g, carbs 4 g, dietary fiber 3 g
Protein 3 g, sodium 23 mg

Savory Muffins

Broccoli Creamed Muffins

Yields 12 | Prep. time 10 minutes | Cooking time 20 minutes

Ingredients
¼ cup heavy whipping cream
1 cup cheddar cheese, shredded
1½ cups broccoli florets
10 large eggs
2 scallions, green and white parts, thinly sliced
¼ teaspoon pepper
1 tablespoon fresh parsley, minced
1 teaspoon onion powder
1 teaspoon salt

Directions
1. Add the broccoli to boiling water in a saucepan and boil for 90 seconds; drain and set aside.
2. Preheat the oven to 400°F (200°C). Grease a 12-cup muffin pan with coconut/avocado oil or cooking spray.
3. In another bowl, beat the eggs and cream. Add the scallions, cheddar, onion powder, salt and pepper. Mix well.
4. Mix in the broccoli florets and parsley.
5. Evenly distribute the batter among the muffin cups.
6. Bake for 15–20 minutes until the eggs are well set.
7. Let cool inside the oven for 5 minutes.
8. Remove from oven and let muffins cool on a wire rack for about 10 minutes.
9. Gently remove muffins from cups; serve fresh.

Spinach Egg Muffins

Yields 12 | Prep. time 10 minutes | Cooking time 15 minutes

Ingredients
10 large eggs
½ teaspoon garlic powder
½ teaspoon dried basil
1–1½ teaspoons salt or to taste
¼–½ teaspoon pepper or to taste
2 cups spinach, chopped
1½ cups grated Parmesan cheese

Directions
1. Preheat the oven to 400°F (200°C). Line a 12-cup muffin pan with paper liners or grease with coconut/olive oil or cooking spray.
2. In another bowl, beat the eggs. Add the salt and pepper. Mix well.
3. Add the garlic powder and basil; mix well.
4. Add the cheese and spinach; mix again.
5. Evenly distribute the batter among the muffin cups.
6. Bake for 12–15 minutes until the eggs are well set.
7. Let cool inside the oven for 5 minutes.
8. Remove from oven and let muffins cool on a wire rack for about 10 minutes.
9. Gently remove muffins from cups; serve fresh.

Avocado Bacon Muffins

Yields 16 | Prep. time 10 minutes | Cooking time 25 minutes

Ingredients
2 tablespoons butter, melted
½ cup almond flour
¼ cup flaxseed meal
5 large eggs
5 slices bacon
2 medium avocados, pitted and halved
4½ ounces Colby Jack cheese, shredded
1 teaspoon dried cilantro
1 teaspoon dried chives
1 teaspoon minced garlic
¼ teaspoon red chili flakes
3 medium spring onions, chopped
Salt and pepper to taste
1½ tablespoons lemon juice
1 teaspoon baking powder
1½ cups coconut milk

Directions
1. Add the bacon to a medium saucepan or skillet and cook over medium heat until evenly crisp and brown. Drain over paper towels and crumble.
2. Preheat the oven to 350°F (175°C). Grease a 12-cup muffin pan with coconut/olive oil or cooking spray.

3. Beat the eggs in a mixing bowl. Add the almond flour, coconut milk, flaxseed meal, spices and lemon juice. Mix well.
4. Add the baking powder, onions and cheese. Mix again.
5. Add the crumbled bacon and butter; mix again.
6. Cut the avocado into small pieces. Mix it in with the bowl mixture.
7. Evenly distribute the batter among the muffin cups.
8. Bake for 25 minutes until well set. Check by inserting a toothpick; if it doesn't come out clean, bake for a few more minutes and repeat.
9. Let cool inside the oven for 5 minutes.
10. Remove from oven and let muffins cool on a wire rack for about 10 minutes.
11. Gently remove muffins from cups; serve fresh.

Nutrition (per muffin)
Calories 144, fat 12 g, carbs 4 g, dietary fiber 2.5 g
Protein 6 g, sodium 481 mg

Bacon Egg Muffins

Yields 12 | Prep. time 10 minutes | Cooking time 20 minutes

Ingredients
½ teaspoon dry mustard powder
Pepper to taste
2 tablespoons fresh parsley or other herbs
8 slices bacon
12 eggs
⅓ cup heavy cream
2 green onions, chopped
3½ ounces cheddar cheese, shredded

Directions

1. Add the bacon to a medium saucepan or skillet and cook over medium heat until evenly crisp and brown. Drain over paper towels and crumble.
2. Preheat the oven to 375°F (190°C). Grease a 12-cup muffin pan with coconut/olive oil or cooking spray.
3. Beat the eggs in a mixing bowl. Add the cream, dry mustard and pepper; mix well.
4. Add the cheese, bacon and onions evenly over the muffin cups. Sprinkle the parsley on top.
5. Evenly distribute the batter among the muffin cups.
6. Bake for 20–25 minutes until the eggs are well set.
7. Let cool inside the oven for 5 minutes.
8. Remove from oven and let muffins cool on a wire rack for about 10 minutes.
9. Gently take the muffins out of the cups; serve fresh.

Nutrition (per muffin)
Calories 181, fat 15 g, carbs 1 g, dietary fiber 0 g
Protein 9 g, sodium 214 mg

Cheese Parsley Muffins

Yields 6 | Prep. time 10 minutes | Cooking time 20 minutes

Ingredients
½ tablespoon powdered sweetener
¾ cups almond flour
2 tablespoons coconut flour
⅛ teaspoon salt
⅛ teaspoon pepper
¾ teaspoon xanthan gum
1 teaspoon dried parsley
1 cup shredded cheddar cheese

1 egg, whisked
2 tablespoons salted butter, melted
6 tablespoons cream
Parsley for sprinkling

Directions

1. Preheat the oven to 400°F (200°C). Grease a 6-cup muffin pan with coconut/olive oil or cooking spray.
2. Add the dry ingredients to a mixing bowl. Mix well.
3. Mix in the shredded cheese.
4. In another bowl, whisk the egg. Add the cream and butter. Mix well.
5. Combine the mixtures and mix well until no visible lumps remain.
6. Evenly distribute the batter among the muffin cups. Add some parsley on top.
7. Bake for 20 minutes until the muffins turn golden brown. Check by inserting a toothpick; if it doesn't come out clean, bake for a few more minutes and repeat.
8. Let cool inside the oven for 5 minutes.
9. Remove from oven and let muffins cool on a wire rack for about 10 minutes.
10. Gently remove muffins from cups; serve fresh.

Nutrition (per muffin)
Calories 242, fat 20.5 g, carbs 3 g, dietary fiber 2 g
Protein 9 g, sodium 293 mg

Broccoli Cheese Muffins

Yields 12 | Prep. time 10 minutes | Cooking time 15 minutes

Ingredients
½ teaspoon dried thyme
½ teaspoon garlic powder
10 large eggs
1–1½ teaspoons salt or to taste
¼–½ teaspoon pepper or to taste
⅔ cup grated cheddar cheese
1½ cups broccoli, steamed and chopped

Directions
1. Preheat the oven to 400°F (200°C). Line a 12-cup muffin pan with silicone liners or grease with coconut/olive oil or cooking spray.
2. In another bowl, beat the eggs. Add the salt and pepper. Mix well.
3. Add the garlic powder and thyme; mix well.
4. Mix in the broccoli and cheddar cheese.
5. Evenly distribute the batter among the muffin cups until they are about ⅔ full. Add more cheese on top, if desired.
6. Bake for 12–15 minutes until well set.
7. Let cool inside the oven for 5 minutes.
8. Remove from oven and let muffins cool on a wire rack for about 10 minutes.
9. Gently take the muffins out of the cups; serve fresh.

Nutrition (per muffin)
Calories 82, fat 5 g, carbs 1 g, dietary fiber 0 g
Protein 6 g, sodium 94 mg

Best Breakfast Muffins

Yields 12 | Prep. time 15 minutes | Cooking time 20 minutes

Ingredients
2 tablespoons finely chopped onion
12 large eggs
Salt and pepper to taste

Spinach
8 grape or cherry tomatoes, halved
¼ cup mozzarella cheese, shredded
¼ cup fresh spinach, roughly chopped

Bacon
¼ cup cheddar cheese, shredded
¼ cup cooked bacon, chopped

Mushrooms
¼ cup red bell pepper, diced
1 tablespoon fresh parsley, chopped
¼ teaspoon garlic powder or ⅓ teaspoon minced garlic
¼ cup brown mushrooms, sliced

Directions
1. Preheat the oven to 350°F (175°C). Grease a 12-cup muffin pan with coconut/olive oil or cooking spray.
2. Beat the eggs in a mixing bowl. Add the onion, salt and pepper. Mix well.
3. Evenly distribute the batter among the muffin cups until they are about half full.
4. Evenly distribute each topping combination over 4 muffins.
5. Bake for 20 minutes until well set.
6. Let cool inside the oven for 5 minutes.

7. Remove from oven and let muffins cool on a wire rack for about 10 minutes.
8. Gently remove muffins from cups; serve fresh.

Nutrition (per muffin)
Calories 82, fat 5 g, carbs 1 g, dietary fiber 0 g
Protein 6 g, sodium 97 mg

Zucchini Ham Muffins

Yields 12 | Prep. time 10 minutes | Cooking time 35 minutes

Ingredients
4 eggs
⅓ cup sour cream
1 zucchini, grated
3½ ounces Parmesan cheese, grated
5 ounces ham, diced
1 teaspoon baking powder
½ teaspoon salt
½ teaspoon pepper
1 cup almond flour

Directions
1. Preheat the oven to 350°F (175°C). Line a 12-cup muffin pan with parchment paper liners.
2. Add the cheese, ham, zucchini, eggs and sour cream to a mixing bowl. Mix well.
3. To another mixing bowl, add the baking powder, almond flour, salt and pepper. Mix well.
4. Combine the mixtures and mix well until no visible lumps remain.
5. Evenly distribute the batter among the muffin cups.

6. Bake for 35–40 minutes until the muffins turn golden brown. Check by inserting a toothpick; if it doesn't come out clean, bake for a few more minutes and repeat.
7. Let cool inside the oven for 5 minutes.
8. Remove from oven and let muffins cool on a wire rack for about 10 minutes.
9. Gently remove muffins from cups; serve fresh.

Nutrition (per muffin)
Calories 135, fat 9 g, carbs 3 g, dietary fiber 1 g
Protein 9 g, sodium 420 mg

Kale Chives Muffins

Yields 8 | Prep. time 10 minutes | Cooking time 30 minutes

Ingredients
¼ cup chives, finely chopped
½ cup almond or coconut milk
6 eggs
1 cup kale, finely chopped
Salt and pepper to taste
8 slices prosciutto or bacon (optional)

Directions
1. Preheat the oven to 350°F (175°C). Grease an 8-cup muffin pan with coconut/olive oil or cooking spray.
2. Line each cup with a slice of prosciutto or bacon.
3. In another bowl, whisk the eggs. Add the kale and chives. Mix well.
4. Mix in the salt and pepper and almond milk.
5. Evenly distribute the batter among the muffin cups until they are about ⅔ full.

6. Bake for 30 minutes until the eggs are well set and the muffins have risen.
7. Let cool inside the oven for 5 minutes.
8. Remove from oven and let muffins cool on a wire rack for about 10 minutes.
9. Gently remove muffins from cups; serve fresh.

Nutrition (per muffin)
Calories 177, fat 11 g, carbs 7 g, dietary fiber 5 g
Protein 16 g, sodium 485 mg

Jalapeño Cheddar Muffins

Yields 12 | Prep. time 15 minutes | Cooking time 30 minutes

Ingredients
2 medium jalapeños
2 teaspoons baking powder
½ teaspoon salt
½ teaspoon garlic powder
2 cups almond flour
¼ cup coconut flour
1½ cups shredded cheddar cheese (divided)
6 tablespoons butter, melted
¾ cup almond milk, unsweetened
4 large eggs

Directions
1. Preheat the oven to 325°F (160°C). Line a 12-cup muffin pan with parchment paper liners.
2. Slice the jalapeños crosswise into 12 thin pieces. Dice the remainder into small pieces.
3. Add the almond flour, coconut flour, salt, baking powder and garlic powder to a mixing bowl. Mix well.

4. Add 1 cup of the cheese and the diced jalapeños.
5. Add the butter, eggs and almond milk. Mix well.
6. Evenly distribute the batter among the muffin cups. Top with the jalapeño slices and the remaining cheese.
7. Bake for 30–35 minutes until the muffins turn golden brown. Check by inserting a toothpick; if it doesn't come out clean, bake for a few more minutes and repeat.
8. Let cool inside the oven for 5 minutes.
9. Remove from oven and let muffins cool on a wire rack for about 10 minutes.
10. Gently take the muffins out of the cups; serve fresh.

Nutrition (per muffin)
Calories 251, fat 21 g, carbs 6 g, dietary fiber 3 g
Protein 10 g, sodium 266 mg

Asparagus Cheese Muffins

Yields 12 | Prep. time 10 minutes | Cooking time 25 minutes

Ingredients
1 cup asparagus, trimmed and chopped into 1-inch pieces
10 eggs
2 tablespoons olive oil
1 small onion, chopped
½ teaspoon salt (divided)
½ cup chopped parsley
¼ cup plain Greek yogurt
¼ teaspoon pepper
4 ounces goat cheese, crumbled

Directions
1. Preheat the oven to 375°F (190°C). Line a 12-cup muffin pan with parchment paper liners.
2. Heat the olive oil over medium heat in a a medium saucepan or skillet.
3. Add the onion, asparagus and ¼ teaspoon of the salt; stir-cook for 4–5 minutes until softened.
4. Whisk the eggs in a mixing bowl. Add the yogurt, parsley, salt and pepper; mix well.
5. Add the cooked vegetables and mix again.
6. Evenly distribute the batter among the muffin cups. Add the crumbled goat cheese on top.
7. Bake for 25–30 minutes until the eggs are well set.
8. Let cool inside the oven for 5 minutes.
9. Remove from oven and let muffins cool on a wire rack for about 10 minutes.
10. Gently remove muffins from cups; serve fresh.

Nutrition (per muffin)
Calories 108, fat 8 g, carbs 1.5 g, dietary fiber 0.5 g
Protein 7 g, sodium 188 mg

Avocado Mushroom Egg Muffins

Yields 12 | Prep. time 15 minutes | Cooking time 20 minutes

Ingredients
1 avocado, pitted and roughly chopped
10 eggs
3½ ounces champignon mushrooms, roughly chopped
1¾ ounces Parmesan cheese, grated
1¾ ounce cream
1 pinch cayenne pepper (optional)
2 teaspoons black pepper
3 teaspoons salt
1 teaspoon Italian herbs

Directions
1. Preheat the oven to 350°F (175°C). Line a 12-cup muffin pan with parchment paper liners or grease with coconut/olive oil or cooking spray.
2. Add all of the ingredients to a mixing bowl. Mix well.
3. Evenly distribute the batter among the muffin cups.
4. Bake for 20 minutes until the eggs are well set.
5. Let cool inside the oven for 5 minutes.
6. Remove from oven and let muffins cool on a wire rack for about 10 minutes.
7. Gently remove muffins from cups; serve fresh.

Nutrition (per muffin)
Calories 107, fat 8.5 g, carbs 1.5 g, dietary fiber 1 g
Protein 6.5 g, sodium 303 mg

Mushroom Chives Muffins

Yields 8 | Prep. time 15 minutes | Cooking time 18 minutes

Ingredients
1 cup mushrooms, cut into small pieces
6 medium eggs
1½ tablespoons chives, raw and chopped
⅔ cup cheddar cheese, grated
1 tablespoon olive oil
¼ teaspoon sea salt
⅛ teaspoon pepper
Olive oil

Directions
1. Preheat the oven to 360°F (180°C). Grease an 8-cup muffin pan with coconut/olive oil or cooking spray.
2. Heat the olive oil over medium heat in a a medium saucepan or skillet.
3. Add the mushrooms and stir-cook for 7–8 minutes until tender. Set aside.
4. In another bowl, beat the eggs. Add the chives, black pepper, salt and grated cheese. Mix well.
5. Mix in the mushrooms.
6. Evenly distribute the batter among the muffin cups.
7. Bake for 18–20 minutes until the top turns brown.
8. Let cool inside the oven for 5 minutes.
9. Remove from oven and let muffins cool on a wire rack for about 10 minutes.
10. Gently take the muffins out of the cups; serve fresh.

Nutrition (per muffin)
Calories 212, fat 16.5 g, carbs 2 g, dietary fiber 0.5g
Protein 13 g, sodium 266 mg

Cheddar Muffins

Yields 15 | Prep. time 15 minutes | Cooking time 12 minutes

Ingredients
2 tablespoons baking powder
4 eggs
3 cups almond flour
½ teaspoon salt
⅔ cup sour cream
½ cup butter, melted
1½ cups cheddar cheese, shredded

Directions
1. Preheat the oven to 400°F (200°C). Grease a 15-cup muffin pan with coconut/olive oil or cooking spray.
2. Add the almond flour, salt and baking powder to a mixing bowl. Mix well.
3. In another bowl, whisk the eggs. Add the butter and sour cream. Mix well.
4. Combine the mixtures and mix well until no visible lumps remain.
5. Mix in the cheese.
6. Evenly distribute the batter among the muffin cups.
7. Bake for 12 minutes until the muffins turn golden brown. Check by inserting a toothpick; if it doesn't come out clean, bake for a few more minutes and repeat.
8. Let cool inside the oven for 5 minutes.
9. Remove from oven and let muffins cool on a wire rack for about 10 minutes.
10. Gently remove muffins from cups; serve fresh.

Nutrition (per muffin)
Calories 264, fat 24 g, carbs 6 g, dietary fiber 2 g
Protein 9 g, sodium 227 mg

Beef Avocado Muffins

Yields 6 | Prep. time 10 minutes | Cooking time 20 minutes

Ingredients
¼ cup heavy cream
1 avocado, pitted and cubed
6 1¾-ounce beef patties
1½ ounces cheddar cheese, cubed or shredded
2 eggs
Pepper to taste

Directions
1. Preheat the oven to 350°F (175°C). Grease a 6-cup muffin pan with coconut/olive oil or cooking spray.
2. Add one beef patty to each cup, shaping it to cover the entire inside surface.
3. Add the avocado and cheese over the patties.
4. Beat the eggs in a bowl. Add the salt and pepper and heavy cream. Mix well.
5. Evenly distribute the batter among the muffin cups.
6. Bake for 20 minutes until the eggs are set and the top is browned.
7. Let cool inside the oven for 5 minutes.
8. Remove from oven and let muffins cool on a wire rack for about 10 minutes.
9. Gently remove muffins from cups; serve fresh.

Nutrition (per muffin)
Calories 368, fat 30 g, carbs 3 g, dietary fiber 2 g
Protein 21 g, sodium 155 mg

Spinach Zucchini Prosciutto Muffins

Yields 12 | Prep. time 15 minutes | Cooking time 20 minutes

Ingredients
3 garlic cloves, minced
1 bell pepper, finely diced
1 tablespoon olive oil
½ onion, finely diced
¼ cup fresh parsley, roughly chopped
1 cup baby spinach, roughly chopped
Salt and pepper to taste
8 large eggs
2 small zucchinis, thinly sliced
12 slices prosciutto
¼ cup coconut milk or nut milk

Directions
1. Preheat the oven to 350°F (175°C). Grease a 12-cup muffin pan with coconut/olive oil or cooking spray.
2. Line each cup with a slice of prosciutto.
3. Heat the olive oil over medium heat in a a medium saucepan or skillet.
4. Add the onion and garlic and stir-cook for 1 minute until softened.
5. Add the spinach, sweet pepper and parsley; stir-cook for 2 minutes until the spinach wilts.
6. Beat the eggs in a bowl. Add the salt and pepper and coconut milk. Mix well.
7. Add the spinach mixture and zucchini. Mix well.
8. Evenly distribute the batter among the muffin cups.
9. Bake for 20 minutes until the eggs are well set.
10. Let cool inside the oven for 5 minutes.

11. Remove from oven and let muffins cool on a wire rack for about 10 minutes.
12. Gently take the muffins out of the cups; serve fresh.

Nutrition (per muffin)
Calories 107, fat 8 g, carbs 2 g, dietary fiber 1 g
Protein 5 g, sodium 101 mg

Zucchini Bacon Muffins

Yields 8 | Prep. time 15 minutes | Cooking time 30 minutes

Ingredients
2 sprigs fresh thyme
½ cup coconut flour
2 cups grated zucchini
1 green onion, chopped
7 large eggs
4–5 slices bacon, diced
½ teaspoon salt
1 teaspoon ground turmeric
½ tablespoon vinegar
1 teaspoon baking powder

Directions
1. Add the bacon to a medium saucepan or skillet and cook over medium heat until evenly crisp and brown. Drain over paper towels.
2. Preheat the oven to 350°F (175°C). Line an 8-cup muffin pan with parchment paper liners or grease with coconut/olive oil or cooking spray.
3. Add the bacon pieces and other dry ingredients to a mixing bowl. Mix well.

4. In another bowl, beat the eggs. Add the vinegar. Mix well.
5. Combine the mixtures and mix well until no visible lumps remain.
6. Evenly distribute the batter among the muffin cups.
7. Bake for 30 minutes until the muffins turn golden brown. Check by inserting a toothpick; if it doesn't come out clean, bake for a few more minutes and repeat.
8. Let cool inside the oven for 5 minutes.
9. Remove from oven and let muffins cool on a wire rack for about 10 minutes.
10. Gently remove muffins from cups; serve fresh.

Nutrition (per muffin)
Calories 104, fat 7 g, carbs 2.5 g, dietary fiber 1 g
Protein 8 g, sodium 388 mg

SWEET BAKED GOOD RECIPES

Cookies

White Chocolate Coconut Cookies

Yields 24 | Prep. time 15 minutes | Cooking time 15 minutes

Ingredients
1½ cups almond flour
½ cups shredded coconut
¼ teaspoon salt
½ teaspoon baking soda
¾ cup granulated sweetener
1 tablespoon gelatin (optional)
½ cup butter, softened
1 large egg
½ cup finely chopped macadamia nuts
½ teaspoon vanilla extract
⅓ cup white chocolate chips, unsweetened

Directions
1. Preheat the oven to 325°F (160°C). Line two cookie sheets with parchment paper.
2. Add the shredded coconut, almond flour, gelatin, baking soda and salt to a mixing bowl. Mix well.
3. In another bowl, beat the eggs. Add the vanilla extract, butter and sweetener. Mix until well blended and fluffy.
4. Combine the mixtures until smooth and without visible lumps.

5. Mix in the macadamia nuts.
6. Roll into 24 1¼-inch balls. Place on the cookie sheets and gently press to ½ inch thickness.
7. Add the chocolate chips on top and press gently.
8. Bake for 12–15 minutes until golden brown.
9. Remove cookies from oven and let cool for 5–10 minutes.
10. Serve fresh or store in an airtight container.

Nutrition (per cookie)
Calories 243, fat 23 g, carbs 6 g, dietary fiber 4 g
Protein 5 g, sodium 106 mg

Chocolate Chip Cookies

Yields 12 | Prep. time 10 minutes | Cooking time 12 minutes

Ingredients
½ teaspoon baking soda
¼ teaspoon salt
¼ cup granulated sweetener
1 teaspoon baking powder
¼ cup butter, melted
1 large egg, beaten
2 teaspoons vanilla extract
2 cups almond flour
½ cup chocolate chips, unsweetened

Directions
1. Preheat the oven to 325°F (160°C). Line a cookie sheet with parchment paper.
2. In another bowl, beat the eggs. Add the vanilla, butter and sweetener. Mix until well blended and creamy.
3. Add the dry ingredients to a mixing bowl. Mix well.

4. Combine the mixtures until smooth and without visible lumps.
5. Drop spoonfuls of batter onto the cookie sheet, leaving some space between each.
6. Bake for 12–15 minutes until golden brown.
7. Remove cookies from oven and let cool for 5–10 minutes.
8. Serve fresh or store in an airtight container.

Nutrition (per cookie)
Calories 198, fat 17 g, carbs 5 g, dietary fiber 3 g
Protein 5 g, sodium 93 mg

Mint Cream Cookies

Yields 24 | Prep. time 25 minutes | Cooking time 12 minutes

Ingredients
¼ cup unsweetened cacao powder
1 teaspoon baking powder
2¼ cups almond flour
3 tablespoons coconut flour
1½ teaspoons xanthan gum
¼ teaspoon salt
1 teaspoon vanilla extract
4 ounces cream cheese
½ cup unsalted butter, softened (divided)
1 egg
1 cup granulated sweetener (divided)
1 teaspoon peppermint extract

Directions
1. Preheat the oven to 350°F (175°C). Line a cookie sheet with parchment paper.

2. Add the baking powder, cacao powder, almond flour, coconut flour, xanthan gum and salt to a mixing bowl. Mix well.
3. To another bowl, add 6 tablespoons of the butter and ½ cup of the sweetener. Mix until fluffy.
4. Mix in the vanilla extract and eggs.
5. Combine the mixtures until smooth and without visible lumps.
6. Roll the dough between two pieces of wax paper to make a ⅛-inch-thick layer.
7. Use a cookie cutter or drinking glass to cut out as many cookies as you can. Re-roll the remaining dough and repeat. You will get around 48 cookies.
8. Place the cookies on the cookie sheet and bake for 12 minutes until golden brown.
9. Remove cookies from oven and let cool for 5–10 minutes.
10. Add the remaining butter and cream cheese to a mixing bowl. Mix well.
11. Spread the mixture evenly on top of half of the cookies. Place the remaining cookies on top and press gently to make cookie sandwiches.
12. Serve fresh or store in an airtight container.

Nutrition (per cookie)
Calories 120, fat 11.5 g, carbs 4 g, dietary fiber 2 g
Protein 3 g, sodium 87 mg

Cinnamon Snicker Doodle Cookies

Yields 16 | Prep. time 10 minutes | Cooking time 15 minutes

Ingredients
Cookies
½ teaspoon baking soda
2 cups almond flour
¾ cup granulated sweetener
½ cup salted butter, softened
Pinch of salt

Coating
1 teaspoon ground cinnamon
2 tablespoons granulated sweetener

Directions
1. Preheat the oven to 350°F (175°C). Line a cookie sheet with parchment paper.
2. Add the cookie ingredients to a mixing bowl. Mix well until a smooth dough forms.
3. Prepare 16 balls from the dough.
4. Combine the sweetener and cinnamon on a plate. Roll each ball to coat evenly.
5. Place the balls on the cookie sheet and flatten them gently with your palm.
6. Bake for 15 minutes until golden brown.
7. Remove cookies from oven and let cool for 5–10 minutes.
8. Serve fresh or store in an airtight container.

Nutrition (per cookie)
Calories 131, fat 13 g, carbs 2.5 g, dietary fiber 1 g
Protein 3 g, sodium 65 mg

Carrot Walnut Cookies

Yields 12 | Prep. time 10 minutes | Cooking time 15 minutes

Ingredients
¼ cup butter, melted
¾ cup granulated sweetener
1 large egg
¼ teaspoon salt
1 teaspoon maple extract
¼ teaspoon baking soda
¾ cup almond flour
¼ cup coconut flour
⅓ cup walnuts, chopped
¼ cup shredded carrots, chopped

Directions
1. Preheat the oven to 350°F (175°C). Line a cookie sheet with parchment paper.
2. Add the baking soda, almond flour, coconut flour and salt to a mixing bowl. Mix well.
3. To another bowl, add the sweetener and melted butter. Mix well.
4. Add the egg and maple extract; mix again.
5. Combine the mixtures into a smooth dough without visible lumps.
6. Mix in the carrots and walnuts.
7. Drop 12 spoonfuls of batter onto the cookie sheet, leaving some space between each.
8. Gently flatten with your palm.
9. Bake for 12–14 minutes until golden brown.
10. Remove cookies from oven and let cool for 5–10 minutes.
11. Serve fresh or store in an airtight container in the refrigerator for up to 2 weeks.

Nutrition (per cookie)
Calories 113, fat 10 g, carbs 3.5 g, dietary fiber 2 g
Protein 3 g, sodium 94 mg

Pine Nut Cookies

Yields 20 | Prep. time 10 minutes | Cooking time 12 minutes

Ingredients
2 cups blanched almond flour
1 cup granulated sweetener
⅓ cup pine nuts
1 large egg
1 teaspoon almond extract
Pinch of salt

Directions
1. Preheat the oven to 325°F (160°C). Line a cookie sheet with parchment paper.
2. In another bowl, beat the eggs. Add the almond extract, salt and sweetener. Mix until well blended and glossy.
3. Add the flour and mix into a stiff dough. Add some water if dough is too dry.
4. Prepare 20 1-inch balls. Place them over the baking sheet and press gently to flatten.
5. Gently press the nuts into the cookies.
6. Bake for 12 minutes until golden brown.
7. Remove cookies from oven and let cool for 5–10 minutes.
8. Serve fresh or store in an airtight container for up to 1 week in the refrigerator and up to 6 months in the freezer.

Nutrition (per cookie)
Calories 83, fat 7 g, carbs 2 g, dietary fiber 1 g
Protein 3 g, sodium 81 mg

Cheesecake Cookies

Yields 22 | Prep. time 10 minutes | Cooking time 13 minutes

Ingredients
½ cup granulated erythritol
1 teaspoon vanilla extract
4 ounces cream cheese, room temperature
½ cup butter
1 teaspoon minced lemon zest

<u>Dry</u>
½ teaspoon salt
1¾ cups almond flour

Directions
1. Preheat the oven to 350°F (175°C). Line a cookie sheet with parchment paper.
2. Add the cream cheese, butter and sugar to a mixing bowl. Mix well.
3. Mix in the vanilla extract.
4. In another bowl, combine the flour and salt.
5. Combine the mixtures until smooth and without visible lumps.
6. Drop spoonfuls of batter onto the cookie sheet, leaving some space between each.
7. Bake for 12 minutes until golden brown.
8. Remove cookies from oven and let cool for 10 minutes.
9. Serve fresh or store in an airtight container.

Nutrition (per cookie)
Calories 105, fat 10 g, carbs 2 g, dietary fiber 1 g
Protein 2 g, sodium 106 mg

Chocolate Fudge Cookies

Yields 10 | Prep. time 10 minutes | Cooking time 12 minutes

Ingredients
¼ cup butter
2 large egg
½ cup granulated sweetener
½ cup unsweetened cocoa powder
1 teaspoon vanilla extract
1 teaspoon baking powder
1 cup almond flour
1 pinch salt

Directions
1. Preheat the oven to 350°F (175°C). Line a cookie sheet with parchment paper.
2. Add the cocoa powder and sweetener to a mixing bowl. Mix well.
3. Mix in the butter.
4. In another bowl, beat the eggs. Add the vanilla and baking powder. Mix well.
5. Combine the mixtures until smooth and without visible lumps.
6. Drop spoonfuls of batter onto the cookie sheet, leaving some space between each.
7. Bake for 12–15 minutes until golden brown.
8. Remove cookies from oven and let cool for 5–10 minutes.
9. Serve fresh or store in an airtight container in the freezer for up to 2–3 months.

Nutrition (per cookie)
Calories 132, fat 11.5 g, carbs 5 g, dietary fiber 3 g
Protein 4.5 g, sodium 78 mg

Classic Shortbread Cookies

Yields 16 | Prep. time 15 minutes |
Cooking time 15–25 minutes

Ingredients
1 pinch salt
1 teaspoon vanilla extract
2 cups almond flour
⅓ cup erythritol
½ cup butter, unsalted and softened
1 large egg

Directions
1. Preheat the oven to 300°F (150°C). Line a cookie sheet with parchment paper.
2. Add the erythritol, almond flour, salt and vanilla to a mixing bowl. Mix well.
3. In another bowl, beat the egg. Add the butter. Mix well.
4. Combine the mixtures into a smooth dough without visible lumps.
5. Roll the dough into small balls and press onto the cookie sheet.
6. Bake for 13–15 minutes until golden brown.
7. Remove cookies from oven and let cool for 5–10 minutes.
8. Serve fresh or store in an airtight container.

Nutrition (per cookie)
Calories 126, fat 12 g, carbs 2 g, dietary fiber 1 g
Protein 3 g, sodium 6 mg

Pumpkin Cheese Cookies

Yields 15 | Prep. time 10 minutes | Cooking time 20 minutes

Ingredients
Dough
⅓ cup pumpkin puree
1 large egg
¾ cup granulated sweetener
6 tablespoons butter, softened
2 cups almond flour
½ teaspoon baking powder
¼ teaspoon ground nutmeg
⅛ teaspoon ground allspice
1 teaspoon ground cinnamon
Pinch of salt

Filling
1 large egg
2 tablespoons granulated sweetener
4 ounces cream cheese
½ teaspoon vanilla extract

Directions
1. Preheat the oven to 350°F (175°C). Line a cookie sheet with parchment paper.
2. Add the dough ingredients to a mixing bowl. Mix into a smooth batter.
3. Drop spoonfuls of batter onto the cookie sheet, leaving some space between each.

4. Using the back of a spoon, round up each drop and make a dent on top.
5. In another bowl, beat the eggs. Add the vanilla, cream cheese and sweetener. Mix well or blend with a blender.
6. Pour a little of the mixture over each dent.
7. Bake for 20 minutes until golden brown.
8. Remove cookies from oven and let cool for 5–10 minutes.
9. Serve fresh or store in an airtight container for up to 1 week in the refrigerator and up to 3 months in the freezer.

Nutrition (per cookie)
Calories 159, fat 15 g, carbs 4 g, dietary fiber 2 g
Protein 5 g, sodium 32 mg

Peanut Butter Cookies

Yields 12 | Prep. time 10 minutes | Cooking time 12 minutes

Ingredients
1 large egg
2 tablespoons almond flour
¾ cup peanut butter
¼ cup granulated sweetener
1 teaspoon vanilla extract (optional)

Directions
1. Preheat the oven to 350°F (175°C). Line a cookie sheet with parchment paper.
2. Add all of the ingredients to a mixing bowl. Mix into a smooth dough.
3. Roll the dough into a thick layer between two pieces of wax paper.

4. Use a cookie cutter or drinking glass to cut out as many cookies as you can. Re-roll the remaining dough and repeat. You will get around 12 cookies.
5. Place the cookies on the cookie sheet.
6. Bake for 12 minutes until golden brown.
7. Remove cookies from oven and let cool for 5–10 minutes.
8. Serve fresh or store in an airtight container.

Nutrition (per cookie)
Calories 108, fat 9 g, carbs 4 g, dietary fiber 1 g
Protein 5 g, sodium 79 mg

Ginger Cookies

Yields 40 | Prep. time 20 minutes | Cooking time 12 minutes

Ingredients
1 tablespoon ground ginger
¼ teaspoon ground cloves
1 teaspoon ground cinnamon
2 cups almond flour
2 tablespoons gelatin
½ teaspoon baking soda
½ cup butter, softened
2 large eggs
½ cup almond butter
1 cup granulated sweetener
½ teaspoon vanilla extract

Directions
1. Preheat the oven to 325°F (160°C). Line two cookie sheets with parchment paper.
2. Add the gelatin, ginger, almond flour, baking soda, cinnamon and cloves to a mixing bowl. Mix well.

3. To another bowl, add the butter, almond butter and sweetener. Mix until smooth.
4. Mix in the vanilla extract and eggs.
5. Combine the mixtures until smooth and without visible lumps.
6. Roll into 1-inch balls and place them on the baking sheets.
7. Bake for 5 minutes; remove baking sheets from oven and press cookies gently with the palm of your hand.
8. Bake for 7 more minutes until evenly brown.
9. Remove cookies from oven and let cool for 5–10 minutes.
10. Serve fresh or store in an airtight container.

Nutrition (per cookie)
Calories 78, fat 6 g, carbs 2 g, dietary fiber 1 g
Protein 2.5 g, sodium 11 mg

Pecan Cookies

Yields 20 | Prep. Time 10 minutes | Cooking time 18 minutes

Ingredients
1¾ cups almond flour
2 tablespoons coconut flour
½ teaspoon vanilla extract
½ cup unsalted butter, softened
½ cup granulated sweetener
½ teaspoon salt
½ cup chopped pecans, toasted

Directions
1. Preheat the oven to 325°F (160°C). Line two cookie sheets with parchment paper.

2. Add the vanilla extract, almond flour, coconut flour and salt to a mixing bowl. Mix well.
3. Mix in the pecans.
4. To another bowl, add the butter and sweetener. Mix until fluffy.
5. Mix in the vanilla extract and eggs.
6. Combine the mixtures until smooth and without visible lumps.
7. Roll into 1-inch balls and place them on the baking sheets. Press gently with the palm of your hand.
8. Bake for 5 minutes; remove the baking sheets and flatten the cookies again till ¼ inch thick.
9. Bake for 10–12 more minutes until evenly brown.
10. Remove cookies from oven and let cool for 5–10 minutes.
11. Serve fresh or store in an airtight container.

Nutrition (per cookie)
Calories 121, fat 11 g, carbs 2.5 g, dietary fiber 1.5g
Protein 2.5 g, sodium 176 mg

Lemon Cardamom Cookies

Yields 16 | Prep. time 10 minutes | Cooking time 15 minutes

Ingredients
2 cups almond flour
½ cup granulated sweetener
6 tablespoons butter, melted
¼ teaspoon ground cardamom
¼ teaspoon clementine or lemon zest
2 ounces dark chocolate (90% or more)

Directions

1. Preheat the oven to 350°F (175°C). Line a cookie sheet with parchment paper.
2. Add the sweetener, cardamom, butter, almond flour and zest to a mixing bowl. Mix into a smooth dough. Refrigerate for 10 minutes.
3. Roll the dough between two pieces of wax paper to make a ½-inch-thick layer.
4. Cut the layer into 16 3×1-inch rectangles. Poke some holes in them with a fork (optional).
5. Place the cookies on the cookie sheet.
6. Bake for 14–15 minutes until golden brown.
7. Remove cookies from oven and let cool for 5–10 minutes.
8. Melt the chocolate in the microwave until fully melted (about 1 minute). Dip the bottom half of each cookie in the melted chocolate. Set aside for a while until chocolate is firm.
9. Serve fresh or store in an airtight container.

Nutrition (per cookie)

Calories 124, fat 11 g, carbs 2.5 g, dietary fiber 0.5g
Protein 4 g, sodium 17 mg

Chocolate Coated Cookies

Yields 10 | Prep. time 20 minutes | Cooking time 30 minutes

Ingredients
¼ cup almond butter
1½ cups almond flour
2 tablespoons powdered sweetener
1 large egg
2–3 teaspoons vanilla extract
1 tablespoon coconut butter
1 tablespoon coconut oil
1 teaspoon baking powder
3¼ ounces dark chocolate (90%)
Pinch of salt

Directions
1. Preheat the oven to 285°F (140°C). Line a baking dish with parchment paper.
2. Add the sweetener, vanilla, ground almonds, baking powder and salt to a mixing bowl. Mix well.
3. In another bowl, beat the eggs. Add the coconut oil, coconut butter and almond butter. Mix well.
4. Combine the mixtures into a smooth dough without visible lumps.
5. Cover with plastic wrap and refrigerate for 30 minutes.
6. Roll the dough between two pieces of wax paper to make a ½-inch-thick layer.
7. Use a cookie cutter or drinking glass to cut out as many 2½-inch cookies as you can. Re-roll the remaining dough and repeat. You will get around 10 cookies.
8. Place the cookies on the baking tray and bake for 30 minutes until golden brown.
9. Remove cookies from oven and let cool for 5–10 minutes.

10. Melt the chocolate in a microwave or in a heat-safe bowl over boiling water.
11. Coat half of each cookie with melted chocolate. Set aside for a while until chocolate is firm.
12. Serve fresh or store in an airtight container for up to 1 week at room temperature and up to 6 months in the freezer.

Nutrition (per cookie)
Calories 211, fat 19 g, carbs 6.5 g, dietary fiber 3 g
Protein 6 g, sodium 87 mg

Bacon Chocolate Cookies

Yields 12 | Prep. time 10 minutes | Cooking time 10 minutes

Ingredients
6 slices bacon
½ cup unsweetened cocoa powder
1 cup chunky peanut butter, unsweetened
1 cup granulated sweetener
1 teaspoon baking soda
1 large egg
1½ teaspoons vanilla extract

Directions
1. Add the bacon to a medium saucepan or skillet and cook over medium heat until evenly crisp and brown. Drain over paper towels and crumble.
2. Preheat the oven to 350°F (175°C). Line a cookie sheet with parchment paper.
3. Add the sweetener, peanut butter and egg to a mixing bowl. Mix well.
4. To another bowl, add the vanilla extract, cocoa powder and baking soda. Mix well.

5. Combine the mixtures until smooth and without visible lumps.
6. Mix in the crumbled bacon.
7. Make 12 pieces from the dough. Place them over the cookie sheet and flatten gently.
8. Bake for 10 minutes until golden brown.
9. Remove cookies from oven and let cool for 5–10 minutes.
10. Serve fresh or store in an airtight container.

Nutrition (per cookie)
Calories 158, fat 13 g, carbs 6 g, dietary fiber 2.5 g
Protein 7 g, sodium 69 mg

Lemon Poppy Seed Cookies

Yields 8 | Prep. time 20 minutes | Cooking time 20 minutes

Ingredients
Cookies
3 tablespoons poppy seeds
1 cup almond flour
¼ cup coconut flour
⅛ teaspoon salt
1 teaspoon baking powder
6 ounces cream cheese, softened
1 large egg
½ cup granulated sweetener
2 tablespoons lemon juice
Zest of 1 lemon
¼ teaspoon liquid stevia extract

Glaze (optional)
2–3 tablespoons lemon juice
¼ cup granulated sweetener

Directions

1. Preheat the oven to 325°F (160°C). Line a cookie sheet with parchment paper.
2. Add the poppy seeds, baking powder, almond flour, coconut flour and salt to a mixing bowl. Mix well.
3. In another bowl, beat the eggs. Add the lemon zest, lemon juice, cream cheese, sweetener and stevia. Mix well.
4. Combine the mixtures into a smooth dough without visible lumps.
5. Make 8–10 balls from the dough. Place them on the cookie sheet and flatten gently.
6. Bake for 20 minutes until golden brown.
7. Remove cookies from oven and let cool for 5–10 minutes.
8. Add the glaze ingredients to a mixing bowl. Mix well.
9. Drizzle the glaze evenly over the cookies. Serve fresh or store in an airtight container.

Nutrition (per cookie)

Calories 189, fat 15 g, carbs 7.5 g, dietary fiber 3.5g
Protein 6 g, sodium 185 mg

Coconut Macaroons

*Yields 10 | Prep. time 10–15 minutes |
Cooking time 8 minutes*

Ingredients
1 tablespoon vanilla extract
1 tablespoon coconut oil, melted
3 egg whites
¼ cup organic almond flour
2 tablespoons granulated sweetener
½ cup shredded coconut

Directions
1. Preheat the oven to 400°F (200°C). Grease a baking sheet with coconut/olive oil or cooking spray.
2. Add the flour, coconut and sweetener to a mixing bowl. Mix well.
3. Mix in the coconut oil and vanilla.
4. In another bowl, whisk the eggs. Add to the flour mixture. Mix until smooth and without visible lumps.
5. Add 10 spoonfuls of the mixture to the baking sheet.
6. Bake for 25 minutes until top becomes golden brown.
7. Remove from oven and let cool completely on a wire rack.
8. Serve fresh.

Nutrition (per serving)
Calories 46, fat 5 g, carbs 1 g, dietary fiber 0.5 g
Protein 2 g, sodium 18 mg

Bars and Squares

Lemon Bars

Serves 8 | Prep. time 15 minutes | Cooking time 45 minutes

Ingredients
1 cup powdered erythritol (divided)
½ cup butter, melted
1¾ cups almond flour (divided)
3 medium lemons
3 large eggs
Pinch of salt

Directions
1. Preheat the oven to 350°F (175°C). Line an 8×8-inch baking pan with parchment paper.
2. Add the salt and butter to a mixing bowl along with ¼ cup of the erythritol and 1 cup of the almond flour. Mix well.
3. Add the mixture to the pan and press to make an even layer.
4. Bake for 20 minutes.
5. Remove from oven and let cool for 10 minutes.
6. In another bowl, beat the eggs. Add the lemon juice and zest as well as the remaining flour and erythritol. Mix well.
7. Pour the mixture over the baked crust and bake for 25 more minutes.
8. Remove from oven and let cool completely on a wire rack.
9. Slice to make square bars. Sprinkle with more erythritol if desired.
10. Serve fresh.

Coconut Caramel Bars

Serves 16 | Prep. time 15 minutes | Cooking time 30 minutes

Ingredients
Crust
¼ cup granulated sweetener
¼ teaspoon salt
1¼ cups almond flour
¼ cup butter, melted

Filling
2 tablespoons coconut oil or butter
4 ounces unsweetened dark chocolate, chopped

Caramel Filling
½ cup granulated sweetener
1½ cups shredded coconut, toasted
3 tablespoons butter
½ teaspoon vanilla extract
¼ teaspoon salt
¾ cup heavy whipping cream

Directions
1. Preheat the oven to 325°F (160°C). Grease an 8×4-inch baking pan with coconut/olive oil or cooking spray.
2. Add the almond flour, sweetener and salt to a mixing bowl. Mix well.
3. Mix in the butter.

94

4. Add the mixture to the baking pan and gently press it into the bottom.
5. Bake for 15–18 minutes until the edges turn golden brown.
6. Remove from oven and let cool completely on a wire rack.
7. Place the coconut oil and chocolate in a heat-safe bowl and microwave for 30 seconds to melt, stirring halfway through.
8. Spread ⅔ of the mixture over the crust to make a chocolate layer.
9. Heat the butter and sweetener over medium heat in a medium saucepan or skillet.
10. Boil for 3–5 minutes until melted and well mixed.
11. Remove from heat; mix in the vanilla, salt and cream.
12. Mix in the coconut.
13. Spread evenly over the chocolate layer.
14. Let cool for 1 hour and slice to make square bars.
15. Drizzle the remaining chocolate over the bars. Serve fresh.

Nutrition (per serving)
Calories 216, fat 21 g, carbs 6.5 g, dietary fiber 3 g
Protein 3 g, sodium 308 mg

Chocolate Peanut Butter Bars

Serves 8 | Prep. time 10 minutes | Cooking time 25 minutes

Ingredients
Base Layer
1½ tablespoons coconut flour
½ cup unsweetened peanut butter
1½ tablespoons granulated sweetener

<u>Top Layer</u>
1 tablespoon unsweetened cocoa powder
½ cup peanut butter
1½ tablespoons powdered erythritol
1½ tablespoons coconut flour

Directions
1. Preheat the oven to 350°F (175°C). Line a baking pan with parchment paper.
2. Add the top layer ingredients to a mixing bowl. Mix well.
3. To another mixing bowl, add the base layer ingredients. Mix well.
4. Add the base layer mixture to the pan and press to make an even layer.
5. Add the top layer mixture; press again.
6. Bake for 25 minutes until the edges turn golden brown.
7. Remove from oven and let cool completely on a wire rack.
8. Slice to make square bars.
9. Serve fresh.

Nutrition (per serving)
Calories 211, fat 15.5 g, carbs 6 g, dietary fiber 4 g
Protein 3 g, sodium 23 mg

Pumpkin Seed Coconut Bars

Serves 10 | Prep. time 10 minutes | Cooking time 15 minutes

Ingredients
2 cups unsweetened finely shredded coconut, toasted
1½ cups pumpkin seeds, toasted
2 eggs
¼ cup + 1 tablespoon granular sweetener
2 tablespoons full-fat butter
1 tablespoon coconut oil
¼ teaspoon salt

Directions
1. Preheat the oven to 350°F (175°C). Line an 8×8-inch baking pan with parchment paper.
2. Add the sweetener to a blender or food processor and blend until powdered.
3. Add the coconut, pumpkin seeds and sweetener powder to a mixing bowl. Mix well.
4. In another bowl, beat the eggs. Add the coconut oil, salt and butter. Mix well.
5. Combine the mixtures and mix well.
6. Add the mixture to the pan and press to make an even layer.
7. Bake for 15 minutes until the edges turn golden brown.
8. Remove from oven and let cool completely on a wire rack.
9. Slice to make square bars.
10. Serve fresh or store in an airtight container in the refrigerator for up to 5 days.

Nutrition (per serving)
Calories 213, fat 18 g, carbs 10.5 g, dietary fiber 7.5g, Protein 7.5 g, sodium 169 mg

Shortbread Pecan Bars

Serves 12 | Prep. time 10 minutes | Cooking time 20 minutes

Ingredients
Crust
3 tablespoons honey
⅓ cup coconut oil or butter, melted
1 cup coconut flour

Topping
5 tablespoons sugar-free maple syrup or stevia drops
½ cup coconut oil
⅔ cup granulated sweetener
2 cups pecans
¼ teaspoon salt

Directions
1. Preheat the oven to 350°F (175°C). Line an 8×8-inch baking pan with parchment paper.
2. Add the coconut flour, syrup and butter/coconut oil to a mixing bowl. Mix until firm and crumbly.
3. Add the mixture to the pan and press to make an even layer.
4. Bake for 10–12 minutes until the edges turn golden brown.
5. Remove from oven and let cool completely on a wire rack.
6. Heat the coconut oil over medium heat in a medium saucepan or skillet.
7. Add the salt and sweetener and stir-cook until bubbly.
8. Mix in the pecans and cook for 1 minute. Remove from heat.
9. Add the pecan mixture over the baked crust.
10. Bake for 5 more minutes.

11. Remove from oven and let cool completely on a wire rack.
12. Refrigerate for 1 hour or until firm. Slice and serve fresh.

Nutrition (per serving)
Calories 132, fat 12 g, carbs 7 g, dietary fiber 4 g
Protein 3 g, sodium 85 mg

Pumpkin Squares

Serves 16 | Prep. time 10 minutes | Cooking time 30 minutes

Ingredients
2 tablespoons avocado oil
¼ cup granulated sweetener
½ cup pumpkin puree
1 teaspoon vanilla extract
2 eggs
1¼ cups almond flour
½ teaspoon salt
1½ teaspoons pumpkin pie spice
1 teaspoon baking soda

Directions
1. Preheat the oven to 350°F (175°C). Line an 8×8-inch baking pan with parchment paper.
2. Add the pumpkin spice, almond flour, salt and baking soda to a mixing bowl. Mix well.
3. In another bowl, beat the eggs. Add the oil, pumpkin puree, sweetener and vanilla extract. Mix well.
4. Combine the mixtures until smooth and without visible lumps.
5. Add the mixture to the pan and press to make an even layer.

6. Bake for 25–30 minutes until the top starts to get dark and the center is baked well.
7. Remove from oven and let cool completely on a wire rack.
8. Slice to make squares.
9. Serve fresh or store in an airtight container in the refrigerator for up to 5 days.

Nutrition (per serving)
Calories 91, fat 7 g, carbs 3.5 g, dietary fiber 1 g
Protein 3 g, sodium 23 mg

Chocolate Chips Walnut Bars

Serves 24 | Prep. time 10 minutes | Cooking time 30 minutes

Ingredients
½ cup unsalted butter
8 ounces cream cheese
2 cups granulated sweetener
5 eggs
1 cup almond flour
⅓ cup coconut flour
2 teaspoons vanilla extract
¼ teaspoon salt
1½ teaspoons baking powder
½ teaspoon xanthan gum (optional)
1 cup chopped walnuts
1 cup unsweetened chocolate chips

Directions
1. Preheat the oven to 350°F (175°C). Line a 12×16-inch baking sheet with parchment paper.
2. Add the butter, cream cheese, sweetener and vanilla to a mixing bowl. Mix well.

3. In another bowl, beat the eggs. Add to the butter mixture. Mix well.
4. In another bowl, add the baking powder, almond flour, coconut flour, salt and xanthan gum. Mix well.
5. Combine the mixtures and mix in the chocolate chips and walnuts.
6. Add the mixture to the baking sheet and press to make an even layer.
7. Bake for 30–35 minutes until the edges turn golden brown.
8. Remove from oven and let cool completely on a wire rack.
9. Slice to make square bars.
10. Serve fresh or store in an airtight container in the refrigerator for up to 5 days.

Nutrition (per serving)
Calories 140, fat 13.5 g, carbs 3 g, dietary fiber 1 g
Protein 4 g, sodium 69 mg

Chia Seed Coconut Bars

Serves 6 | Prep. time 10 minutes | Cooking time 45 minutes

Ingredients
1 tablespoon coconut oil
1 cup unsweetened shredded dried coconut
¼ cup chia seeds
½ cup water
1 tablespoon granulated sweetener
½ cup cashews
¼ teaspoon vanilla extract

Directions

1. Add the water and chia seeds to a bowl. Soak for 15 minutes; drain and set aside.
2. Preheat the oven to 350°F (175°C). Line a 9×9-inch baking pan with parchment paper.
3. Add the shredded coconut, coconut oil, chia seeds, vanilla extract and sweetener to a mixing bowl. Mix well.
4. Mix in the cashews.
5. Add the mixture to the pan and press to make an even layer ¾ inch thick.
6. Bake for 45 minutes until the edges turn golden brown.
7. Remove from oven and let cool completely on a wire rack.
8. Slice to make square bars.
9. Serve fresh.

Nutrition (per serving)

Calories 164, fat 14 g, carbs 9.5 g, dietary fiber 6 g

Protein 4 g, sodium 38 mg

Cardamom Walnut Balls

Yields 18–20 | Prep. time 10 minutes |
Cooking time 18 minutes

Ingredients
2 tablespoons coconut flour
1 teaspoon baking powder
2 cups almond flour
1 cup finely chopped walnuts
¾ teaspoon coarsely ground cardamom
¼ teaspoon salt
½ cup granulated sweetener
½ cup butter, softened
1 large egg
¼ teaspoon stevia extract
1 teaspoon vanilla extract
¾ cup powdered sweetener

Directions
1. Preheat the oven to 325°F (160°C). Line two baking sheets with parchment paper.
2. Add the cardamom, almond flour, walnuts, coconut flour, baking powder and salt to a mixing bowl. Mix well.
3. In another bowl, beat the eggs. Add the butter and granulated sweetener. Mix until fluffy and well blended.
4. Mix in the vanilla.
5. Combine the mixtures until smooth and without visible lumps.
6. Prepare ¾-inch balls from the mixture.
7. Place them over the baking sheets.
8. Bake for 18–20 minutes until golden brown.
9. Remove from oven and let cool completely on a wire rack.

10. Add the powdered sweetener to a mixing bowl. Coat the walnut balls evenly with the sweetener.
11. Serve fresh.

Nutrition (per ball)
Calories 170, fat 16 g, carbs 5 g, dietary fiber 2 g
Protein 5 g, sodium 117 mg

Cakes and Rolls

Pumpkin Cake

Serves 8 | Prep. time 15 minutes | Cooking time 30 minutes

Ingredients
4 large eggs
½ tablespoon unsalted butter, softened
1 cup pumpkin puree
1½ teaspoons granulated sweetener
¼ cup unsalted butter, melted
¼ teaspoon salt
1 teaspoon vanilla extract
1 teaspoon pumpkin pie spice
1 teaspoon baking soda
2 cups blanched finely ground almond flour

Directions
1. Preheat the oven to 350°F (175°C). Grease a 9-inch cake pan with some butter.
2. Whisk the eggs in a bowl. Add the butter, sweetener, pumpkin puree, vanilla and salt. Mix well.
3. Add the pumpkin pie spice, almond flour and baking soda to a mixing bowl. Mix well.
4. Combine the mixtures and mix well into a smooth, thick mixture with no visible lumps.
5. Add to the pan and smooth the top surface with a spatula or spoon.
6. Bake for 30–35 minutes until the edges turn golden brown. Check by inserting a toothpick; if it doesn't come out clean, bake for a few more minutes and repeat.
7. Remove pan from oven and let cake cool completely on a wire rack.

8. Slice and serve fresh.

Nutrition (per serving)
Calories 266, fat 23 g, carbs 9 g, dietary fiber 4 g
Protein 9 g, sodium 240 mg

Cinnamon Tea Cake

Serves 8 | Prep. time 15 minutes | Cooking time 20 minutes

Ingredients
Batter
2 eggs
1 teaspoon vanilla essence
3½ ounces unsalted butter, softened
¼ cup granulated sweetener
1 teaspoon baking powder
1¼ cups almond flour
¼ cup unsweetened almond milk

Topping
1 tablespoon granulated sweetener
1 teaspoon cinnamon
2 tablespoons unsalted butter, melted

Directions
1. Preheat the oven to 340°F (170°C). Grease an 8-inch cake pan with some butter or line it with parchment paper.
2. To make the batter, add the sweetener and butter to a mixing bowl. Mix well until smooth and creamy.
3. In another bowl, whisk the eggs. Add to the butter mixture. Mix well.
4. Add the remaining batter ingredients to a mixing bowl. Mix well.

5. Combine the mixtures and mix well into a smooth, thick mixture with no visible lumps.
6. Add the mixture to the pan and smooth the top surface with a spatula or spoon.
7. Bake for 20–25 minutes until the edges turn golden brown. Check by inserting a toothpick; if it doesn't come out clean, bake for a few more minutes and repeat.
8. Remove pan from oven and let cake cool completely on a wire rack.
9. To make the topping, add the sweetener and cinnamon to a mixing bowl. Mix well.
10. Brush the cake with the melted butter and sprinkle the cinnamon mixture on top.
11. Slice and serve fresh.

Nutrition (per serving)
Calories 232, fat 22 g, carbs 3.5 g, dietary fiber 2 g
Protein 5 g, sodium 28 mg

Chocolate Zucchini Cake

Serves 12 | Prep. time 10 minutes | Cooking time 30 minutes

Ingredients
¼ cup almond milk
1 cup shredded zucchini
4 eggs
½ cup butter, melted
⅓ cup coconut flour
1 cup almond flour
½ cup cocoa powder
1 teaspoon baking powder
½ cup granulated sweetener

Chocolate Ganache
3 tablespoons butter
¼ cup almond milk
7 ounces dark chocolate

Directions

1. Preheat the oven to 360°F (180°C). Grease an 8×8 cake pan with some butter.
2. Add the cocoa powder, sweetener, almond flour, coconut flour and baking powder to a mixing bowl. Mix well.
3. In another bowl, beat the eggs. Add the almond milk and butter. Mix well.
4. Combine the mixtures until smooth and without visible lumps. Mix in the zucchini.
5. Add the mixture to the pan and smooth the top surface with a spatula or spoon.
6. Bake for 30–40 minutes until the edges turn golden brown. Check by inserting a toothpick; if it doesn't come out clean, bake for a few more minutes and repeat.
7. Remove pan from oven and let cake cool completely on a wire rack.
8. Add all of the ganache ingredients to a mixing bowl. Mix gently and microwave for 2 minutes until chocolate melts completely.
9. Spread the chocolate frosting over the cake.
10. Slice and serve fresh.

Nutrition (per serving)
Calories 197, fat 12 g, carbs 9 g, dietary fiber 2.5 g
Protein 4 g, sodium 76 mg

Chocolate Cake

Serves 8 | Prep. time 10 minutes |
Cooking time 14–15 minutes

Ingredients
¼ cup cocoa powder
2 tablespoons Dutch cocoa or regular cocoa powder
2¼ teaspoons baking powder
1½ cups fine almond flour
½ teaspoon salt
⅓ cup water or coconut milk
3 eggs
1½ teaspoons vanilla extract
⅓ cup granulated sweetener

Directions
1. Preheat the oven to 350 degrees F (175°C). Line an 8-inch cake pan with parchment paper.
2. Add all the ingredients except for the eggs to a mixing bowl. Mix well.
3. In another bowl, beat the eggs.
4. Combine the mixtures until smooth and without visible lumps.
5. Add the mixture to the pan and smooth the top with a spatula or spoon.
6. Bake for 14–15 minutes until the top turns golden brown. Check by inserting a toothpick; if it doesn't come out clean, bake for a few more minutes and repeat.
7. Remove from oven and let cake cool completely on a wire rack.
8. Slice and serve fresh.

Nutrition (per serving)
Calories 130, fat 9 g, carbs 6 g, dietary fiber 3.5 g
Protein 7 g, sodium 175 mg

Blueberry Cake

Serves 12 | Prep. time 10 minutes | Cooking time 35 minutes

Ingredients
1 tablespoon lemon juice
¼ cup almond flour
½ cup coconut flour
3 cups frozen blueberries, thawed
¼ teaspoon salt
½ cup granulated sweetener
1 teaspoon ground cinnamon
1 teaspoon baking powder
½ cup melted butter or coconut oil

Directions
1. Preheat the oven to 375°F (190°C). Grease an 8×8-inch cake pan with coconut/olive oil or cooking spray.
2. Add the sweetener, blueberries and lemon juice to a mixing bowl. Mix well.
3. Pour the mixture into the cake pan.
4. Add the baking powder, coconut flour, almond flour, cinnamon and salt to a mixing bowl. Mix well.
5. Pour the flour mixture over the blueberry layer. Pour the melted butter on top.
6. Bake for 30–35 minutes until the top turns golden brown. Check by inserting a toothpick; if it doesn't come out clean, bake for a few more minutes and repeat.
7. Remove from oven and let cake cool completely on a wire rack.
8. Slice and serve fresh.

Nutrition (per serving)
Calories 199, fat 18 g, carbs 9 g, dietary fiber 2 g
Protein 2 g, sodium 41 mg

Cream Cheese Butter Cake

Serves 10 | Prep. time 10 minutes | Cooking time 35 minutes

Ingredients
Base
1 teaspoon baking powder
3 tablespoons coconut flour
¼ cup powdered sweetener
1 tablespoon beef gelatin (optional)
½ cup butter
½ teaspoon vanilla extract
2 large eggs

Top Layer
8 ounces cream cheese
½ cup butter
½ teaspoon vanilla extract
50 drops liquid stevia
¼ cup powdered erythritol
2 large eggs

Directions
Base
1. Preheat the oven to 350°F (175°C). Grease an 8-inch springform pan with coconut/olive oil or cooking spray.
2. In another bowl, beat the eggs. Add the butter and vanilla. Mix well.
3. Add the coconut flour, erythritol, baking powder and gelatin to a mixing bowl. Mix well.

Top Layer
1. Add the butter and cream cheese to a mixing bowl. Mix well.
2. Mix in the erythritol, stevia, vanilla extract and eggs until smooth.

<u>Cake</u>
1. Add the flour mixture to the pan and smooth the top with a spatula or spoon.
2. Pour in the top layer and smooth the surface again.
3. Bake for 30–35 minutes until the sides turn golden brown. Check by inserting a toothpick; if it doesn't come out clean, bake for a few more minutes and repeat.
4. Remove from oven and let cake cool completely on a wire rack.
5. Slice and serve fresh.

Nutrition (per serving)
Calories 295, fat 30 g, carbs 2 g, dietary fiber 0 g
Protein 5 g, sodium 305 mg

Lemon Cheesecake

Serves 12 | Prep. time 10 minutes | Cooking time 60 minutes

Ingredients
6 tablespoons butter
¾ cup granulated sweetener
6 eggs
1 cup cream cheese
¼ cup lemon juice
1 tablespoon baking powder
2½ cups almond flour
½ cup coconut flour
2 teaspoons lemon zest

Lemon Glaze
2 teaspoons water
1 tablespoon butter
1 teaspoon lemon extract or zest
½ cup powdered sweetener

Directions
1. Preheat the oven to 350°F (175°C). Line an 8×8-inch cake pan with parchment paper.
2. Add the cream cheese, sweetener and butter to a mixing bowl or food processor. Mix until smooth.
3. In another bowl, beat the eggs. Add the flours, lemon juice, baking powder and zest. Mix well.
4. Combine the mixtures until smooth and without visible lumps.
5. Add the mixture to the pan and smooth the top with a spatula or spoon.
6. Bake for 60–70 minutes until the edges turn golden brown. Check by inserting a toothpick; if it doesn't come out clean, bake for a few more minutes and repeat.

7. Remove from oven and let cake cool completely on a wire rack.
8. In another bowl, combine all of the glaze ingredients.
9. Spread glaze evenly on top of the cake.
10. Slice and serve fresh.

Nutrition (per serving)
Calories 322, fat 28 g, carbs 10 g, dietary fiber 5 g
Protein 10 g, sodium 168 mg

Carrot Cake

Serves 8 | Prep. time 15 minutes | Cooking time 25 minutes

Ingredients
½ teaspoon baking soda
½ teaspoon nutmeg
1 teaspoon cinnamon
1½ cups almond flour
½ teaspoon salt
3 eggs
¼ cup sugar-free maple-flavored syrup or granulated sweetener
1 cup finely shredded carrots
½ cup pecans, chopped
2 tablespoons coconut oil

Directions
1. Preheat the oven to 350°F (175°C). Line an 8×8-inch baking pan with parchment paper.
2. Add the baking soda, almond flour, salt, cinnamon and nutmeg to a mixing bowl. Mix well.
3. In another bowl, beat the eggs. Add the sweetener and coconut oil. Mix well.
4. Combine the mixtures until smooth and without visible lumps.
5. Mix in the carrots and pecans.
6. Add the mixture to the pan and press to make an even layer.
7. Bake for 25–27 minutes until the edges turn golden brown.
8. Remove from oven and let cool completely on a wire rack.
9. Slice to make square bars.
10. Serve fresh or store in an airtight container in the refrigerator for up to 5 days.

Nutrition (per serving)
Calories 235, fat 18 g, carbs 5 g, dietary fiber 2.5 g
Protein 7 g, sodium 221 mg

Sweet Muffins

Chocolate Muffins

Yields 12 | Prep. time 10 minutes | Cooking time 20 minutes

Ingredients
½ cup granulated erythritol
1½ teaspoons baking powder
1 cup almond flour
½ cup unsweetened cocoa powder
1 teaspoon vanilla extract
3 large eggs
⅔ cup heavy cream
3 ounces unsalted butter, melted
½ cup unsweetened chocolate chips

Directions
1. Preheat the oven to 350°F (175°C). Line a 12-cup muffin pan with cupcake papers.
2. Add the cocoa powder, almond flour, erythritol and baking powder to a mixing bowl.
3. Add the eggs, vanilla extract and heavy cream. Mix well until no visible lumps remain.
4. Add the melted butter and continue to mix.
5. Add the chocolate chips and mix again.
6. Evenly distribute the prepared batter among the muffin cups.
7. Bake for 20 minutes until golden brown. Check by inserting a toothpick; if it doesn't come out clean, bake for a few more minutes and repeat.
8. Let cool inside the oven for 5 minutes.
9. Remove from oven and let muffins cool on a wire rack for about 10 minutes.

10. Gently take the muffins out of the cups; serve fresh.

Nutrition (per muffin)
Calories 212, fat 20 g, carbs 8 g, dietary fiber 5 g
Protein 5 g, sodium 27 mg

Blueberry Muffins

Yields 12 | Prep. time 20 minutes | Cooking time 25 minutes

Ingredients
1 tablespoon baking powder
1 teaspoon salt
1 teaspoon baking soda
3 cups almond flour
¼ cup coconut flour
7 tablespoons coconut oil
¾ cup granulated sweetener
½ cup applesauce, unsweetened
2 teaspoons vanilla extract
3 large eggs
⅔ cup fresh blueberries

Directions
1. Preheat the oven to 350°F (175°C). Grease a 12-cup muffin pan with coconut/olive oil or cooking spray.
2. Add the coconut flour, almond flour, baking powder, salt and baking soda to a mixing bowl. Mix well.
3. In another bowl, beat the eggs. Add the sweetener, applesauce, coconut oil and vanilla. Mix well.
4. Combine the mixtures and mix well until no visible lumps remain.
5. Mix in the blueberries and set aside for 5 minutes.

6. Bake for 23–25 minutes until the muffins turn golden brown. Check by inserting a toothpick; if it doesn't come out clean, bake for a few more minutes and repeat.
7. Let cool inside the oven for 5 minutes.
8. Remove pan from oven and let muffins cool for 15–20 minutes on the counter.
9. Gently take the muffins out of the cups; serve fresh.

Nutrition (per muffin)
Calories 247, fat 22 g, carbs 9.5 g, dietary fiber 4 g
Protein 7.5 g, sodium 218 mg

Banana Walnut Muffins

Yields 10 | Prep. time 10 minutes | Cooking time 20 minutes

Ingredients
2 tablespoons ground flaxseed (optional)
2 teaspoons baking powder
1¼ cups almond flour
½ cup powdered erythritol
5 tablespoons butter, melted
½ teaspoons ground cinnamon
2½ teaspoons banana extract
1 teaspoon vanilla extract
¼ cup sour cream
¼ cup almond milk, unsweetened
2 eggs

Topping
¾ cup chopped walnuts
1 tablespoon almond flour
1 tablespoon butter, cold
1 tablespoon powdered erythritol

Directions

1. Preheat the oven to 350°F (175°C). Line a standard muffin pan with 10 parchment paper liners.
2. Add the almond flour, baking powder, ground flaxseed, cinnamon and erythritol to a mixing bowl. Mix well.
3. Add the vanilla extract, butter, banana extract, almond milk and sour cream.
4. Mix well. Add the eggs and mix well until no visible lumps remain.
5. Evenly distribute the batter among the muffin cups.
6. In a food processor, chop the walnuts, butter and almond flour into small pieces. Add more butter if the mixture is too dry.
7. Sprinkle the nut mixture over the batter evenly and press down gently. Sprinkle powdered erythritol on top.
8. Bake for 20 minutes until the muffins turn golden brown. Check by inserting a toothpick; if it doesn't come out clean, bake for a few more minutes and repeat.
9. Let cool inside the oven for 5 minutes.
10. Remove pan from oven and let muffins cool on a wire rack for about 20–30 minutes.
11. Gently remove muffins from cups; serve fresh.

Nutrition (per muffin)

Calories 248, fat 22 g, carbs 7 g, dietary fiber 3 g
Protein 7 g, sodium 91 mg

Poppy Seed Lemon Muffins

Yields 12 | Prep. time 10 minutes | Cooking time 20 minutes

Ingredients
⅓ cup erythritol
1 teaspoon baking powder
¾ cup almond flour
¼ cup golden flaxseed meal
2 tablespoons poppy seeds
¼ cup heavy cream
¼ cup salted butter, melted
3 large eggs
3 tablespoons lemon juice
Zest of 2 lemons
1 teaspoon vanilla extract
25 drops liquid stevia

Directions
1. Preheat the oven to 350°F (175°C). Grease a 12-cup muffin pan with coconut/olive oil or cooking spray.
2. Add the almond flour, flaxseed meal, poppy seeds and erythritol to a mixing bowl. Mix well.
3. Add the eggs, butter and heavy cream. Mix well until no visible lumps remain.
4. Mix in the vanilla extract, baking powder, liquid stevia, lemon zest and lemon juice.
5. Evenly distribute the batter among the muffin cups.
6. Bake for 18–20 minutes until the muffins turn golden brown. Check by inserting a toothpick; if it doesn't come out clean, bake for a few more minutes and repeat.
7. Let cool inside the oven for 5 minutes.
8. Remove from oven and let muffins cool on a wire rack for about 10 minutes.
9. Gently remove muffins from cups; serve fresh.

Classic Keto Muffins

Yields 12 | Prep. time 10 minutes | Cooking time 20 minutes

Ingredients
2 ounces cream cheese, softened
2 tablespoons butter, softened
⅓ cup granular sweetener
½ cup unsweetened vanilla almond milk
4 eggs
2 teaspoons vanilla
1 cup almond flour
½ cup coconut flour
¼ teaspoon salt
1 teaspoon baking powder

Topping
2 tablespoons coconut flour
1 cup almond flour
¼ cup granular sweetener
¼ cup butter, softened
1 teaspoon cinnamon
½ teaspoon molasses (optional)

Directions
1. Preheat the oven to 350°F (175°C). Line a 12-cup muffin pan with parchment paper liners.
2. Add the batter ingredients to a blender or food processor and blend until well combined.
3. Evenly distribute the batter among the muffin cups.

4. Add the topping ingredients to a blender or food processor and blend until crumbs form.
5. Sprinkle the topping over the batter in the muffin cups.
6. Bake for 20–25 minutes until the muffins turn golden brown. Check by inserting a toothpick; if it doesn't come out clean, bake for a few more minutes and repeat.
7. Let cool inside the oven for 5 minutes.
8. Remove from oven and let muffins cool on a wire rack for about 10 minutes.
9. Gently remove muffins from cups; serve fresh.

Nutrition (per muffin)
Calories 222, fat 18 g, carbs 9 g, dietary fiber 4 g
Protein 7 g, sodium 156 mg

Cinnamon Keto Muffins

Yields 12 | Prep. time 10 minutes | Cooking time 25 minutes

Ingredients
½ cup granular erythritol
2½ cups almond flour
2 teaspoons baking powder
3 large eggs
1 teaspoon cinnamon
⅓ cup almond milk
½ cup full-fat sour cream
1 teaspoon vanilla
⅓ cup unsalted butter, melted

Topping
1 tablespoon granular erythritol
¼ teaspoon cinnamon

Directions

1. Preheat the oven to 350°F. Line a 12-cup muffin pan with parchment paper liners.
2. Add the almond flour, erythritol, cinnamon and baking powder to a mixing bowl. Mix well.
3. In another bowl, beat the eggs. Add the milk, butter, sour cream and vanilla. Mix well.
4. Combine the mixtures and mix well until no visible lumps remain.
5. Evenly distribute the batter among the muffin cups.
6. In another bowl, combine all of the topping ingredients. Sprinkle the topping evenly over the batter in the muffin cups.
7. Bake for 22–25 minutes until the muffins turn golden brown. Check by inserting a toothpick; if it doesn't come out clean, bake for a few more minutes and repeat.
8. Let cool inside the oven for 5 minutes.
9. Remove from oven and let muffins cool on a wire rack for about 10 minutes.
10. Gently remove muffins from cups; serve fresh.

Nutrition (per muffin)

Calories 241, fat 21 g, carbs 6 g, dietary fiber 3 g
Protein 7 g, sodium 32 mg

Pumpkin Cinnamon Muffins

Yields 20 | Prep. time 10 minutes | Cooking time 15 minutes

Ingredients
1 tablespoon cinnamon
½ cup almond flour
1 teaspoon baking powder
½ cup nut butter (almond, peanut etc.)
½ cup coconut oil
½ cup pumpkin puree

Glaze
¼ cup almond or coconut milk
¼ cup coconut butter
1 tablespoon granulated sweetener
2 teaspoons lemon juice

Directions
1. Preheat the oven to 350°F (175°C). Line a 12-cup muffin pan with parchment paper liners.
2. Add the dry ingredients to a mixing bowl. Mix well.
3. To another mixing bowl, add the butter, coconut oil and pumpkin puree. Mix well.
4. Combine the mixtures and mix well until no visible lumps remain.
5. Evenly distribute the batter among the muffin cups.
6. Bake for 10–15 minutes until the muffins turn golden brown. Check by inserting a toothpick; if it doesn't come out clean, bake for a few more minutes and repeat.
7. Let cool inside the oven for 5 minutes.
8. Remove from oven and let muffins cool on a wire rack for about 10 minutes.
9. In another bowl, combine all of the glaze ingredients.

10. Gently remove muffins from cups. Drizzle with glaze. Set aside until they firm up. Serve fresh.

Nutrition (per muffin)
Calories 112, fat 9 g, carbs 3 g, dietary fiber 2 g
Protein 5 g, sodium 64 mg

Blackberry Muffins

Yields 10 | Prep. time 10 minutes | Cooking time 25 minutes

Ingredients
2½ cups blanched almond flour, finely ground and sifted
⅓ cup granulated sweetener
¼ teaspoon salt
1½ teaspoons baking powder
⅓ cup unsweetened almond or cashew milk
⅓ cup coconut oil or melted butter
½ teaspoon vanilla extract
3 large eggs
¾ cup blackberries or raspberries, fresh or frozen and thawed

Directions
1. Preheat the oven to 350°F (175°C). Line a 12-cup muffin pan with 10 parchment paper liners.
2. Add the granulated sweetener, almond flour, baking powder and salt to a mixing bowl. Mix well.
3. Mix in the berries.
4. In another bowl, beat the eggs. Add the vanilla extract, coconut oil or butter and almond milk. Mix well.
5. Combine the mixtures and mix well until no visible lumps remain.
6. Evenly distribute the batter among the muffin cups.

7. Bake for 25 minutes until the muffins turn golden brown. Check by inserting a toothpick; if it doesn't come out clean, bake for a few more minutes and repeat.
8. Let cool inside the oven for 5 minutes.
9. Remove pan from oven and let muffins cool on a wire rack.
10. Gently remove muffins from cups; serve fresh.

Nutrition (per muffin)
Calories 277, fat 25 g, carbs 8 g, dietary fiber 3 g
Protein 8 g, sodium 101 mg

Apple Spice Muffins

Yields 12 | Prep. time 10 minutes | Cooking time 25 minutes

Ingredients
1 teaspoon baking powder
1 teaspoon ground cinnamon
½ teaspoon salt
2½ cups almond flour
¾ cup granulated stevia or erythritol
4 large eggs
¼ cup butter or coconut oil, melted
¼ cup unsweetened almond milk
1 teaspoon vanilla extract
1 small (4 ounces) Granny Smith apple, peeled, seeded and finely diced

Directions
1. Preheat the oven to 350°F (175°C). Grease a 12-cup muffin pan with coconut/olive oil or cooking spray.

2. Add the almond flour, baking powder, sweetener, cinnamon and salt to a mixing bowl. Mix well.
3. Add the butter or coconut oil. Mix again.
4. In another bowl, beat the eggs. Add the almond milk and vanilla. Mix well.
5. Combine the mixtures and mix well until no visible lumps remain.
6. Mix in the diced apple.
7. Evenly distribute the batter among the muffin cups.
8. Bake for 25–30 minutes until the muffins turn golden brown. Check by inserting a toothpick; if it doesn't come out clean, bake for a few more minutes and repeat.
9. Let cool inside the oven for 5 minutes.
10. Remove from oven and let muffins cool on a wire rack for about 10 minutes.
11. Gently remove muffins from cups; serve fresh.

Nutrition (per muffin)
Calories 198, fat 17 g, carbs 7 g, dietary fiber 3 g
Protein 7 g, sodium 185 mg

Carrot Cake Muffins

Yields 12 | Prep. time 10 minutes | Cooking time 45 minutes

Ingredients
1 teaspoon baking powder
1 teaspoon cinnamon
1 cup almond flour
½ cup granular sweetener
½ teaspoon salt
3 small carrots, shredded
¾ cup olive oil
2 eggs, beaten

Frosting
2 tablespoons butter, room temperature
4 ounces cream cheese, room temperature
¼ cup powdered sweetener
½ teaspoon vanilla extract
¼ teaspoon almond extract
2 tablespoons heavy whipping cream
4 drops liquid stevia

Directions
1. Preheat the oven to 350°F (175°C). Line a 12-cup muffin pan with parchment paper liners.
2. Add the almond flour, baking powder, sweetener, cinnamon and salt to a mixing bowl. Mix well.
3. In another bowl, beat the eggs. Add the carrots and olive oil. Mix well.
4. Combine the mixtures and mix well until no visible lumps remain.
5. Evenly distribute the batter among the muffin cups.
6. Bake for 40–45 minutes until the muffins turn golden brown. Check by inserting a toothpick; if it doesn't come out clean, bake for a few more minutes and repeat.

7. Let cool inside the oven for 5 minutes.
8. Remove from oven and let muffins cool on a wire rack for about 10 minutes.
9. Gently remove muffins from cups. Set aside.
10. To make the frosting, add the butter and cream cheese to a mixing bowl. Mix well.
11. Add the heavy cream, sweetener, vanilla, almond and stevia and mix well.
12. Pour the frosting over the muffins. Serve fresh or refrigerate until frosting has firmed up.

Nutrition (per muffin)
Calories 251, fat 25 g, carbs 5 g, dietary fiber 2 g
Protein 4 g, sodium 196 mg

Pumpkin Cheese Muffins

Yields 12 | Prep. time 10 minutes | Cooking time 20 minutes

Ingredients
4 large eggs
½ cup butter, softened
⅔ cup + 1 tablespoon granulated erythritol
¾ cup pumpkin puree
1 teaspoon vanilla extract
4 teaspoons baking powder
2 teaspoons pumpkin spice
1½ cups almond flour
½ cup coconut flour
½ teaspoon salt
8 ounces cream cheese, softened

Directions

1. Preheat the oven to 350°F (175°C). Grease a 12-cup muffin pan with coconut/olive oil or cooking spray.
2. Add the butter and ⅔ cup erythritol to a mixing bowl. Mix until fluffy.
3. In another bowl, beat the eggs. Add the butter mixture, pumpkin puree and vanilla. Mix well.
4. Add the baking powder, almond flour, coconut flour, pumpkin spice and salt to a mixing bowl. Mix well.
5. Combine the mixtures and mix well until no visible lumps remain.
6. Evenly distribute the batter among the muffin cups.
7. Add the 1 tablespoon erythritol and softened cream cheese to a mixing bowl. Mix well.
8. Drop a spoonful of the mixture over each muffin and spread evenly.
9. Bake for 20–25 minutes until the muffins turn golden brown. Check by inserting a toothpick; if it doesn't come out clean, bake for a few more minutes and repeat.
10. Let cool inside the oven for 5 minutes.
11. Remove from oven and let muffins cool on a wire rack for about 10 minutes.
12. Gently remove muffins from cups; serve fresh.

Nutrition (per muffin)

Calories 261, fat 23 g, carbs 6 g, dietary fiber 4 g
Protein 7 g, sodium 623 mg

Zucchini Spice Muffins

Yields 8 | Prep. time 10 minutes | Cooking time 25 minutes

Ingredients
1 cup grated zucchini
⅓ cup coconut oil
6 medium eggs
¾ cup coconut flour
¼ cup granulated sweetener
½ teaspoon baking soda
1 teaspoon cinnamon
¼ teaspoon nutmeg, grated
4 drops stevia liquid

Directions
1. Preheat the oven to 350°F (175°C). Line a 12-cup muffin pan with 8 parchment paper liners.
2. Heat the oil over medium heat in a medium saucepan or skillet.
3. Add the zucchini and stir-cook until well mixed with the oil.
4. Add all the ingredients except for the zucchini to a mixing bowl. Mix well.
5. Add the cooked zucchini.
6. Mix well until no visible lumps remain.
7. Evenly distribute the batter among the muffin cups.
8. Bake for 25 minutes until the muffins turn golden brown. Check by inserting a toothpick; if it doesn't come out clean, bake for a few more minutes and repeat.
9. Let cool inside the oven for 5 minutes.
10. Remove from oven and let muffins cool on a wire rack for about 10 minutes.
11. Gently remove muffins from cups; serve fresh.

Nutrition (per muffin)
Calories 175, fat 13 g, carbs 6.5 g, dietary fiber 4 g
Protein 5.5 g, sodium 68 mg

Super Strawberry Muffins

Yields 12 | Prep. time 10 minutes | Cooking time 20 minutes

Ingredients
⅓ cup unsweetened vanilla almond milk
3 large eggs
½ cup granular erythritol
⅓ cup coconut oil
2½ cups almond flour
2 teaspoons baking powder
1 cup strawberries, fresh or thawed

Directions
1. Preheat the oven to 350°F (175°C). Line a 12-cup muffin pan with parchment paper liners or grease with coconut/olive oil or cooking spray.
2. Add the baking powder and almond flour to a mixing bowl. Mix well.
3. In another bowl, whisk the eggs. Add the almond milk, sweetener and coconut oil. Mix well.
4. Combine the mixtures and mix well until no visible lumps remain.
5. Mix in the strawberries.
6. Evenly distribute the batter among the muffin cups.
7. Bake for 22–25 minutes until the muffins turn golden brown. Check by inserting a toothpick; if it doesn't come out clean, bake for a few more minutes and repeat.
8. Let cool inside the oven for 5 minutes.

9. Remove pan from oven and let muffins cool on a wire rack for about 30–60 minutes.
10. Gently remove muffins from cups; serve fresh.

Nutrition (per muffin)
Calories 207, fat 19 g, carbs 6.5 g, dietary fiber 2.5g, Protein 6.5 g, sodium 97 mg

Applesauce Spice Up Muffins

Yields 12 | Prep. time 10 minutes | Cooking time 20 minutes

Ingredients
3 large eggs, whisked
3 cups almond flour
½ cup ghee, melted
1 teaspoon baking soda
1 teaspoon nutmeg
¼ teaspoon cloves
3 tablespoons cinnamon
¼ cup applesauce
1 teaspoon lemon juice
Stevia to taste

Directions
1. Preheat the oven to 350°F (175°C). Grease a 12-cup muffin pan with coconut/olive oil or cooking spray.
2. Add the dry ingredients to a mixing bowl. Mix well.
3. In another bowl, beat the eggs. Add the applesauce, ghee and lemon juice. Mix well.
4. Combine the mixtures and mix well until no visible lumps remain.
5. Evenly distribute the batter among the muffin cups.

6. Bake for 18–20 minutes until the muffins turn golden brown. Check by inserting a toothpick; if it doesn't come out clean, bake for a few more minutes and repeat.
7. Let cool inside the oven for 5 minutes.
8. Remove from oven and let muffins cool on a wire rack for about 10 minutes.
9. Gently remove muffins from cups; serve fresh.

Nutrition (per muffin)
Calories 241, fat 22 g, carbs 7 g, dietary fiber 4 g
Protein 7 g, sodium 52 mg

Avocado Chocolate Muffins

Yields 10 | Prep. time 15 minutes | Cooking time 25 minutes

Ingredients
Dry Ingredients
1 cup almond flour
⅓ cup coconut flour
½ cup granular sweetener
1 teaspoon cinnamon
1 teaspoon baking soda
2 teaspoons cream of tartar
⅓ cup unsweetened cocoa powder
⅓ cup dark chocolate, roughly chopped

Wet Ingredients
4 large eggs
2 tablespoons coconut milk or heavy cream
2 medium avocados, peeled, seeded and halved
15–20 drops stevia liquid

Directions

1. Preheat the oven to 350°F (175°C). Line a standard muffin pan with 10 parchment paper liners.
2. Add the avocado halves to a blender or food processor until smooth.
3. Add the other wet ingredients and blend until smooth.
4. Add the dry ingredients except for the chocolate to a mixing bowl. Mix well.
5. Add the avocado mixture. Mix well until no visible lumps remain.
6. Mix in the chocolate pieces, reserving some for topping.
7. Evenly distribute the batter among the muffin cups. Sprinkle the reserved chocolate pieces on top.
8. Bake for 25 minutes until the muffins turn golden brown and crispy. Check by inserting a toothpick; if it doesn't come out clean, bake for a few more minutes and repeat.
9. Let cool inside the oven for 5 minutes.

Nutrition (per muffin)

Calories 210, fat 16 g, carbs 13.5 g, dietary fiber 7g, Protein 7.5 g, sodium 169 mg

Zucchini Chocolate Muffins

Yields 12 | Prep. time 10 minutes | Cooking time 25 minutes

Ingredients
¼ teaspoon salt
½ teaspoon baking soda
2 cups almond flour (or almond meal)
¼ cup unsweetened cocoa
¼ cup coconut oil
¼ cup granular sweetener
3 large eggs
½ cup sugar free dark chocolate chips (optional)
¾ cup shredded zucchini

Directions
1. Preheat the oven to 350°F (175°C). Line a 12-cup muffin pan with parchment paper liners.
2. Add the almond flour, salt, cocoa and baking soda to a mixing bowl. Mix well.
3. In another bowl, beat the eggs. Add the sweetener and coconut oil. Mix well.
4. Mix in the zucchini and chocolate chips.
5. Combine the mixtures and mix well until no visible lumps remain.
6. Evenly distribute the batter among the muffin cups.
7. Bake for 22–25 minutes until the muffins turn golden brown. Check by inserting a toothpick; if it doesn't come out clean, bake for a few more minutes and repeat.
8. Let cool inside the oven for 5 minutes.
9. Remove from oven and let muffins cool on a wire rack for about 10 minutes.
10. Gently remove muffins from cups; serve fresh.

Nutrition (per muffin)
Calories 247, fat 16 g, carbs 14 g, dietary fiber 7 g
Protein 6 g, sodium 117 mg

Orange Muffins

Yields 6 | Prep. time 10 minutes | Cooking time 30 minutes

Ingredients
2 tablespoons coconut oil
¼ cup fresh orange juice
2 cups almond flour, blanched
3 large eggs
½ teaspoon cardamom
1 teaspoon baking powder
¼ teaspoon sea salt
1 tablespoon orange zest
2 teaspoons stevia powder

Glaze
1 tablespoon coconut oil
½ tablespoon stevia powder
¼ cup coconut butter

Directions
1. For glaze, melt the butter in a saucepan; add the coconut oil and stir until smooth.
2. Remove from heat; mix in the stevia powder. Set aside.
3. Preheat the oven to 350°F (175°C). Line a 6-cup muffin pan with parchment paper liners.
4. Whisk the eggs in a bowl. Add the orange juice and orange zest. Mix well.
5. Add the baking powder, cardamom, almond flour, stevia and salt to a mixing bowl. Mix well.

6.   Combine the mixtures and mix well. Add the coconut oil.
7.   Mix well until no visible lumps remain.
8.   Evenly distribute the batter among the muffin cups.
9.   Bake for 25–30 minutes until the muffins turn golden brown. Check by inserting a toothpick; if it doesn't come out clean, bake for a few more minutes and repeat.
10. Let cool inside the oven for 5 minutes.
11. Remove from oven and let muffins cool on a wire rack for about 10 minutes.
12. Gently remove muffins from cups; drizzle with prepared glaze and serve fresh.

Nutrition (per muffin)
Calories 257, fat 26 g, carbs 11 g, dietary fiber 5 g
Protein 12.5 g, sodium 218 mg

Peanut Butter Cacao Muffins

Yields 6 | Prep. time 20 minutes | Cooking time 25 minutes

Ingredients
1 teaspoon baking powder
1 pinch salt
1 cup almond flour
½ cup granular sweetener
⅓ cup low-carb unsweetened peanut butter
2 large eggs
⅓ cup almond milk
½ cup cacao nibs or unsweetened chocolate chips

Directions

1. Preheat the oven to 350°F (175°C). Grease a 12-cup muffin pan with coconut/olive oil or cooking spray.
2. Add the almond flour, salt, baking powder and sweetener to a mixing bowl. Mix well.
3. In another bowl, beat the eggs. Add the peanut butter and almond milk. Mix well.
4. Combine the mixtures and mix well until no visible lumps remain.
5. Mix in the cacao nibs.
6. Evenly distribute the batter among the muffin cups.
7. Bake for 25–30 minutes until the muffins turn golden brown. Check by inserting a toothpick; if it doesn't come out clean, bake for a few more minutes and repeat.
8. Let cool inside the oven for 5 minutes.
9. Remove from oven and let muffins cool on a wire rack for about 10 minutes.
10. Gently remove muffins from cups; serve fresh.

Nutrition (per muffin)

Calories 265, fat 20.5 g, carbs 4.5 g, dietary fiber 2.5 g, Protein 7.5 g, sodium 210 mg

RECIPE INDEX

APPENDIX

Cooking Conversion Charts

1. Measuring Equivalent Chart

Type	Imperial	Imperial	Metric
Weight	1 dry ounce		28 g
	1 pound	16 dry ounces	0.45 kg
Volume	1 teaspoon		5 ml
	1 dessert spoon	2 teaspoons	10 ml
	1 tablespoon	3 teaspoons	15 ml
	1 Australian tablespoon	4 teaspoons	20 ml
	1 fluid ounce	2 tablespoons	30 ml
	1 cup	16 tablespoons	240 ml
	1 cup	8 fluid ounces	240 ml
	1 pint	2 cups	470 ml
	1 quart	2 pints	0.95 l
	1 gallon	4 quarts	3.8 l
Length	1 inch		2.54 cm

* Numbers are rounded to the closest equivalent

2. Oven Temperature Equivalent Chart

Fahrenheit (°F)	Celsius (°C)	Gas Mark
220	100	
225	110	1/4
250	120	1/2
275	140	1
300	150	2
325	160	3
350	180	4
375	190	5
400	200	6
425	220	7
450	230	8
475	250	9
500	260	

* Celsius (°C) = T (°F)-32] * 5/9
** Fahrenheit (°F) = T (°C) * 9/5 + 32
*** Numbers are rounded to the closest equivalent

Printed in Great Britain
by Amazon